The Treacherous Dichotomy

Physical Illness versus Mental Illness

Stefan Lerner, M.D.

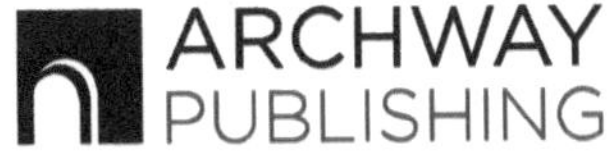

Archway Publishing books may be ordered through booksellers or by contacting:

Archway Publishing
1663 Liberty Drive
Bloomington, IN 47403
www.archwaypublishing.com
1 (888) 242-5904

ISBN: 978-1-4808-7208-0 (sc)
ISBN: 978-1-4808-7209-7 (hc)
ISBN: 978-1-4808-7210-3 (e)

Library of Congress Control Number: 2018965526

Print information available on the last page.

Archway Publishing rev. date: 12/07/2018

AUTHOR'S NOTE

The mission of this book is to promote radical change in the so-called field of mental health. In the process, it is highly critical of the psychiatric profession as a whole, while acknowledging that some psychiatrists maintain high standards of care. If your own psychiatrist has been helpful to you, by all means continue treatment with the doctor. If not, an excellent second opinion can be available at a teaching hospital that has a direct association with a school of medicine. The psychiatric attendings in these institutions generally maintain high standards of care. There is usually one such center in most states.

CONTENTS

PREFACE

Here are some distinctions between therapy psychiatrists and brain psychiatrists. The therapy psychiatrist's practice will fit into a particular pattern. He will see each patient for forty-five minutes at least on a weekly basis for several years. He emphasizes psychotherapy as his primary treatment modality. The psychotherapy is often some derivative of psychoanalysis, according to the individual idiosyncrasies of the psychiatrist. It often will follow no predictable goal-oriented format, and there may be no specific criteria for ending the therapy.

All physicians are required to acquire a certain number of points documenting they have been attending educational conferences, reading professional journals, etc. The therapy psychiatrist will emphasize the practice of psychotherapy as the main focus of this continuing education and will generally steer away from the study of the brain, neuroscience, and complex, sophisticated pharmacology. They consider themselves philosophers of the psyche, the unconscious, and character molding, ultimately creating a new, improved individual. Although the therapy psychiatrist went to medical school, the objective was never to fully identify as a practicing physician; it was to reach a higher earnings tier for their psychotherapeutic services. Therapy psychiatrists constitute approximately 70–80 percent of all psychiatrists.

The brain psychiatrist generally does not do a long-term psychoanalytical psychotherapy. His standard session, hopefully, is twenty-five to thirty minutes and not a five-to-ten-minute med-check. Many psychiatrists, especially younger ones, are forced into the med-check mode by insurance companies. The med-check is inadequate, not providing the time to survey the patient's life for significant stressors or provide explanations for what can be complex pharmacological treatments. Treatment session frequency varies widely, from weekly for very acutely ill patients to three or four appointments per year for stable patients. In his continuing education, he will emphasize brain study, supportive therapy approaches, and details of pharmacological treatments. He adheres closely to the medical model in the same manner as physicians in other specialties like internal medicine, surgery, and cardiology.

Since he does not adhere to the time-consuming routine of regular forty-five-minute psychotherapy sessions, he is much more available to see a greater number of patients than the therapy psychiatrist, with much less expense per patient. He does not negate the need for the standard psychotherapy approach, but refers to therapists for that, who are certified to provide scientifically proven specific forms of therapies like CBT (cognitive behavioral therapy) and RP (response prevention therapy for OCD).

Generally, PhDs have expertise in specialized therapies. Social workers (MSWs) are trained to provide a more general form of psychotherapy—the forty-five-minute weekly session that therapy psychiatrists provide—but on a much more economical basis, not adding financial pressure on top of the symptoms and disabilities of the illnesses.

CHAPTER 1

The Stigma of Mental Illness and the Treacherous Dichotomy

The *treacherous dichotomy* refers to how we categorize human ailments. Out of long habit and for ease of reference, while generally not intending harm consciously, we place them into two discrete groupings: the physical and the mental. We have been referencing diseases in this matter for centuries—since long before the underlying physiological mechanisms came to light. We continue to do so in every aspect of our culture: psychiatry, medicine, the press, literature, media, and educational institutions.

Nearly every informed person would agree that stigmatizing mental illness is undesirable. Over the past half century, there has been some diminishment in the stigma, but the basic tendency remains in force in spite of this half-century effort at destigmatization. The question is if this stigma will ever be eliminated. We need to bring into action the ultimate weapon against this stigma, the elimination of the treacherous dichotomy itself: the very categorization of diseases as physical or mental.

With the enlightenment bestowed upon us by modern neuroscience, we know serious so-called mental illnesses are indeed physical. The mental categorization is totally misleading in addition to conferring the burden of stigmatization. The treacherous dichotomy is like a magnet that attracts and holds metal. If we introduce iron filings onto a paper near a strong magnet, we cannot expect the filings not to be drawn to the magnetic lines of force. Similarly, as long as we categorize certain diseases as mental in our minds, we cannot expect that stereotypical thinking and attitudes toward so-called mental illness will not coalesce in our subconscious minds. Therefore, it is impossible to efficaciously attack the stigma until we abandon the physical-mental dichotomy. In other words, we must no longer call it mental illness. We must eradicate this term when referring to human ailments and diseases.

We can actually categorize the concept of mental illness as a form of a slur, the last in common usage, bandied about in conversation and print as if it was polite terminology. But unlike more neutral words, it immediately attracts to itself like the magnet and iron filings, a constellation of other associated words and attitudes that spring forth in the subconscious and even conscious mind. We all know this is the case as soon as we pay attention to our own subconscious thought processes. This would almost be almost humorous—if it wasn't injurious to so many millions of people.

This raises the issue of what a stereotype is. Stereotypes are the building blocks of stigma. In the case of the so-called mentally ill, the stereotypes always portray them in a negative light and disrespectful tone, especially when contrasted with people who are designated as having physical illnesses like asthma, diabetes, seizures, or heart disease. It is remarkable the number of insulting, disrespectful adjectives the label mentally ill triggers in the mind: insane, bonkers, loco, madman, fruitcake, weird, crazy, nuts, nut job, demented, wacko, schizo, loony, peculiar, and so on.

This litany remains just below the surface, ready to influence our behaviors, reactions, and attitudes toward the so-called mentally ill, often conveying rejection and coolness to them. This emotional distancing from them has real-life manifestations. They will be seen as less-desirable social companions and candidates for friendship. This sets up an undercurrent of a feedback loop where they, as sensitive individuals, sense the emotional distancing and withdraw more emotionally. The ultimate destination of this vicious feedback loop is painful emotional isolation for the so-called mentally ill individual.

There is also overt discrimination occupationally and in housing. The individual labeled mentally ill has internalized the entire litany of negative labels and attitudes. In addition to the symptoms, suffering, and disabilities stemming from the so-called mental illness itself, he suffers an overlay of shame, guilt, humiliation, and loss of self-esteem induced by the suspicion (or reality) of the people he tries to interact with. Below the surface of social veneer, they really do think of him in disparaging ways.

Illusory Correlation

The headline was "In Quest to Explain Shootings, exploring Mental Illness." Included in the article was another heading: "Grim Statistics. Some of the Deadliest US Killing Sprees in the Past Three Decades." Certainly what leaps to mind is that serial murders are committed by the so-called mentally ill. The dramatic headings of shootings and mental illness are linked in the bold print of the headline. One could almost shudder at the prospect of being in the vicinity of someone who has a so-called mental illness. Illusory correlation is a process whereby people misattribute rare behaviors at higher rates to minority group members and overestimate the frequency of the negative behavior in the linked group. It can feel like the so-called mentally ill person can be suspected of being seriously dangerous. This does not lead to a relaxed, amiable environment.

Stereotype Threat

Of course, stereotypes are internalized by those who are stereotyped, and this sensitizes the self-stereotyper to the anticipation of being judged by others along the *lines* of the stereotype. The anticipation of being judged by others according to the content of the stereotype does not lead to a benign sequence of events. The threat of having the stereotype applied to the self has been shown to result in decrements of social and intellectual performance as well as inducing the very behavior predicted by the stereotype. Thus, the stereotype is reinforced in both individuals.

A 1977 study by Snyder, Tanke, and Berscheid found a similar pattern in social interactions between men and women. Male undergraduate students were asked to talk to female undergraduates, whom they believed to be physically attractive or unattractive, on the phone. The conversations were taped, and analysis showed that men who thought they were talking to attractive women communicated in a more positive and friendlier manner than men who believed they were talking to unattractive women. This altered the women's behavior. Female subjects who, unknowingly to them, were perceived to be physically attractive behaved in a friendly, likeable, and sociable manner in comparison with subjects who were regarded as unattractive.

The Physical Nature of Mental Illness

It is bad enough to be afflicted with a dysfunctioning brain striking at the heart of well-being, inverting experience into a dystopian nightmare, ravishing self-esteem, achievement, and success, but then to compound this suffering by attaching the stigmatizing label, mental illness is gratuitously cruel.

The major so-called mental illnesses strike at the most human organ in the body, that organ which is capable of appreciating what is beautiful and splendid. It also can bring forth the experience of great torment and agony. Modern neuroscientific research makes clear that the data are overwhelming that so-called mental illness must be redeposited on the physical part of the ledger along with the neurological brain illnesses like convulsive disorders, myasthenia gravis, and multiple sclerosis. What will be left under the heading of mental disorders? Nothing should be left. The concept is antiquated, outdated, antiscientific, and stigmatizing. The physical nature of so-called mental disorders is manifested at the genetic, cellular, and metabolic levels. Lesions are not visible to the unaided eye, but aren't genes physical? Are abnormal neuronal connections physical? Are abnormal chemicals physical?

It is now the time; the gestalt clamors for change. We must radically rearrange our thinking to be consistent with science. We must decide once and for all there is no such entity as mental illness.

The negativity associated with so-called mental illness, as long as this label persists, serves as deterrence to seeking treatment. It is natural to resist accepting such a label. Even if treatment is finally obtained, compliance with it may be diminished for the same reason. Keeping the category and label of mental illness will greatly increase suffering, interrupt functioning and the prospect of worse disabilities, and enormously increase expense to the health care system. This gratuitous labeling is particularly problematic for the adolescent age group, which is particularly sensitive to stigmatization and humiliation. The cost is delayed entry into treatment or even total resistance to it. Adolescents are particularly susceptible to developmental delays and dysfunctions due to inadequately treated illness, resulting in potentially lifelong suffering and disabilities.

There are difficulties associated with making a major substantive change, but I am going to suggest we start now. We must correct individuals who continue to use the term *mental illness*. We must advise them that science has proven that the major so-called mental illnesses are not mental at all; they are caused by physical abnormalities of the brain. There is no logic whatsoever to separating them by category: mental versus physical illness, neurological illnesses, and kindred brain diseases, which everyone accepts as physical.

We must eliminate the phrase *mental illness* and reference the root psyche as a disease identifier. If neurology uses the root *neuro*, we should too. I declare that psychiatric illness henceforth should be called *neuriatric illness*. I have transitioned from being a psychiatrist to being a *neuriatrist*. In the DSM classification of so-called mental disorders, there are many diagnoses that do not classify as major neuriatric disorders. They should be stripped of the mental label and reclassified as cognitive, behavioral, emotional, and personality dysregulations.

CHAPTER 2

My Patients

Over the years, I've evaluated and treated thousands of patients. It disturbs me that they are forced to identify themselves as mentally ill. They are the ones who made it into treatment; untold others are unable to accept the label and thereby not do not transition to appropriate diagnosis or treatment. I regard the patients I've treated as very fortunate, especially if they have serious so-called mental illnesses, which can cause so much suffering and disability.

I have always participated in continuing education, keeping current in clinical psychopharmacology. The mental health system is a maze of confusing services and varied practitioners. Countless individuals never receive an appropriate diagnosis, differential diagnosis, or sophisticated medical treatment. Clinical psychopharmacology involves an understanding of actual brain mechanisms and which medications may be suitable to ameliorate specific symptoms and dysregulations.

So many of my patients have been gracious, friendly, and personable. What possible benefit can there be to linking them with the stereotypes conjured up by being labeled mentally ill? Suffering and disability do not dichotomize themselves into mental or physical categories. They are erroneously separated from physical illnesses—mental illnesses—and are an equal-opportunity partner when it comes to suffering.

Three Seniors

I first evaluated Mr. Tunis more than a decade ago, when he was sixty-seven. He was the owner of a company he had founded and built. Of particular note was his courtly and gracious manner. He was referred by a psychotherapist for both depression and severe panic attacks persisting in spite of psychotherapy. There was a significant family history in which he described depression on the maternal side. At the time of our first consultation, he was transitioning into retirement and was worried. He said, "What'll I do next?" He was concerned about continuing to be an attentive husband who was sensitive to his wife's needs. He was proud of his family, particularly his grandchildren.

He had experienced a severe panic attack several months prior to our consultation and was constantly in dread of a reoccurrence. On the Hamilton Depression Rating Scale,[1] his seventeen-item subtotal was 20½ (a normal value is 7 or less). This was consistent with major depression of moderate degree. His symptoms included persistent sadness, nagging self-reproach, insomnia in the form of awakening two hours prematurely and being unable to return to sleep, intense worrying, and an unshakable conviction that tormented him that he had a terminal disease. He was started on Effexor, an antidepressant in the SNRI class. A month later, he was much improved; he was no longer in torment and was able to relax about his health. The HAM-D scale score, when readministered, objectively measured his improvement. The score dropped to 7, which was considered a remission of the depressive episode. He also felt secure that additional panic attacks would be prevented.

We continued with Effexor therapy for eleven years. He devised activities to enjoy his retirement and wasn't at all bothered by his

---

[1] This is a test administered by the provider. It consists of a series of standardized questions that can be scored. The total sum of points can be diagnostic for major depression. If the patient's score is 8 or less, he is free of major depression. Mild depression scores 10 to 18. Scores of 18 or higher indicate more severe depression.

previous symptoms. Then he began experiencing symptoms of lightheadedness and dizziness. His cardiologist diagnosed a type of cardiac arrhythmia, and even though it was not proven, he implicated the Effexor, which was then discontinued.

A different antidepressant, Lexapro (Escitalopram), replaced it, but it did not have such a clear-cut benefit. A second antidepressant, mirtazapine, was added (combination therapy), and finally, a third medication, Abilify (Apiprazole), was added for the purpose of augmentation.

Over the ensuing two years, although not feeling as well as previously on the Effexor, he was managing. During the subsequent summer, his suffering amplified. He said, "Severe depression and panic … I cannot lift my spirits … I have feelings of dread … the valley of despair!"

I increased his Lexapro from twenty to thirty milligrams. The Hamilton Depression Rating Scale score had increased to 23. I increased the mirtazapine to forty-five milligrams. There was some alleviation of his anxiety and despair, but the extreme morning dread improved.

He said, "Not the doom and gloom … I feel better … more myself than in several years. The level of improvement is huge. I have been worse this past month."

I broached the option of hospitalization at an excellent tertiary care center for observation, diagnosis, and treatment, but he felt he couldn't go because his family was looking forward to the holidays.

Over the New Year's weekend, he took an overdose of medication and slashed his wrists. He was hospitalized in the local community hospital as an inpatient. He had a course of six electroconvulsive therapy treatments. It's interesting that the hospital staff did not contact the undersigned during the patient's hospitalization and discharged him to the care of a nurse practitioner. There was trouble hooking up with her, and he decided to return to the care of the undersigned and his former therapist.

When seen in mid-May, his symptoms were in remission. The

hospital doctors had replaced the generic Lexapro with Cymbalta while maintaining the mirtazapine and Abilify. Unfortunately, this period of improvement was transitory.

"Pretty bad … Anxiety overtakes me … I toss and turn … I wake up too early."

He was referred back to the community hospital for outpatient electroconvulsive therapy treatments, receiving eight treatments over two months. By early August, he was feeling generally better—more energy, more active—and sleeping soundly.

At the end of August, after the eighth outpatient ECT treatment, he was feeling more withdrawn. He said, "The medication interferes with my motivation." He was spending his days in bed, sinking into despair. "I see no end to it."

An emergency appointment was made, and his wife accompanied him. She was exasperated that he wasn't being more active. "He's not himself … He's staying in his room."

He said, "I can't face life the way I'm doing now."

He agreed to be admitted to the originally recommended tertiary care center, and the undersigned had several communications with the attending psychiatrist there.

He remained there for nearly eight weeks, finally improving after a long course of seventeen right unilateral ECT treatments.

He could not tolerate an older type of antidepressant, a tricyclic, because of orthostatic hypotension. This class of antidepressant occasionally has a special benefit for his subtype of depressive illness, melancholic.

The attending noted the patient's wife did not wish to participate in discussions at the hospital with the professional staff treating her husband, but his son was more agreeable to it.

He had his first follow-up appointment in my office a week after discharge. The undersigned reviewed the course of treatment and his discharge clinical status with the attending psychiatrist at the tertiary care hospital.

This dignified elderly man never appeared to be mentally ill. The severe, recurrent illness that caused so much suffering and disability at his advanced age certainly packed a vicious wallop of symptomatology, although it wasn't visible as an aberration to the unschooled eye. His wife had an expectation he should just sort himself out and get over it. This is not a surprise; she has been conditioned by the pervasive mental/physical dichotomy of classifying illnesses wherein mental illness is reflexively viewed as a lesser category of illness that one can control and overcome if one is determined. This unspoken belief that influenced his wife's view of his illness was an added weight to his suffering.

He could not help—at some subconscious level—agreeing with her. The mental/physical dichotomy exacts an additional burden on those on the mental side of it, including guilt, lowered self-esteem, and a sense of weakness, failure, and disapproval. Indeed, the mental/physical dichotomy is treacherous. It emotionally traumatizes those unfortunate patients classified in the mental categorization of illness.

Two Additional Elderly Patients

Mrs. P and her husband impressed me immediately with their graciousness and warmth.[2] I truly enjoyed their company as we attended to the business of diagnosis, supportive therapy, and pharmacological management. She was in her thirties when she had her first episode of major depression and subsequently had two additional ones. She required hospitalization on each occasion. Since

---

[2] I'm sure that when they entertained friends and family, the latter would look forward to the next social occasion with them; they would look fully at home at a White House dinner. Mrs. P. was also an accomplished fine arts painter in oils. She exhibited in galleries and sold some of her pieces, which were in a realistic or Impressionistic style. She also painted portraits, some from life and others of famous individuals, including scientists such as Einstein and several popes. They also loved to travel, relating their experiences in a number of regions (e.g., Portugal, France, Germany, Eastern Europe, and South America). He was a rose connoisseur. They would both relate how proud they were of their grandchildren.

the last hospitalization, she had been treated with an agent from the older group of antidepressants, Norpramine (desipramine), and a small dosage of a first-generation antipsychotic called Mellaril.

The next years went well. She continued her social life and artistic endeavors. In the fall of her fourth year of uneventful treatment, her husband reported, “Things are going real bad.”

On Monday, she had been wonderful—and then she abruptly accused him of going to whores. She called 911 repeatedly, demanding that the police come. She admitted she had not been taking her medicine. She said, “I don’t need it.”

He contacted the undersigned and was advised that she needed immediate evaluation in the emergency room. She was admitted and had a course of ECT.[3]

A month later, when seen after her discharge, she was her usual pleasant self. Her clinical course was uneventful for an additional five years. Then, prior to Christmas, she started staying in bed and watching religious programs. She admitted, “I’m getting very emotional in church.”

She accepted hospitalization and received five or six ECTs. When seen after discharge, she gave her signature declaration of well-being. “I feel wonderful … I’m not tired … I have much more energy.”

It should not be acceptable that Mrs. B. is pigeonholed in the category of being mentally ill. It is perfectly obvious she is an intelligent, creative person who is pleasant, social, and good-hearted, and she has a pleasing sense of humor. Her episodic symptoms were manifestations of a severe dysregulation of specific brain mechanisms, some understood, many not yet known. This dignified woman does not deserve being stigmatized by the humiliating label mental.

***

Mr. X made a deep impression on me. He was not my private patient. He had been assigned to my care when I was employed on a hospital

[3] Electroconvulsive therapy.

psychiatric unit. It had nothing to do with what he told me—he could not talk—but I learned of his accomplishments from his adult children. He was a veteran of World War II. After the war, he had a family and a successful career as an engineer. Then, in his senior years, he developed a severe vein thrombosis in his leg. He stopped talking, communicating, or caring for himself.

When I first met him, he was seated in a chair and not moving. He did not acknowledge my presence. His eyes were glazed, staring ahead. He was transferred to a psychiatrically supervised medical unit, and I lost contact with him. I always wondered what this previously active, successful veteran of World War II made of his sudden state of complete helplessness and vulnerability. It was such a wrenching twist in the course of his life in its final phase, and he had no chance to prepare for or adjust to it. The random punishment meted out to some unfortunate individuals is ghastly.[4] Perhaps we breathe a sigh of relief that it isn't us, but perhaps it could be? Perhaps we could be labeled mentally ill at some unforeseen future time.

A Married Mother of a Young Son is Tortured

Sarah, when first seen, was married and the mother of a young son. It was clear that she was very intelligent and desperate to gain relief from her symptoms. She had been under treatment with another psychiatrist for four years, but the chart notes were available. She had related her symptoms to him: "It feel like my skin is crawling … intense panic and fear to the point, I feel crazy at times."

Her mother had said, "Sarah, this is not you; something is happening to you."

During our interview, Sarah said, "It's extraordinarily painful … I feel intense pressure. I want it to stop."

She originally went to the psychiatrist after she called her ob-gyn, describing her symptoms and saying, "I'm in serious trouble."

The psychiatrist prescribed Pamelor (Nortriptyline). After

[4] By what we characterize as episodes of mental illness.

starting it, she called a day later complaining of anxiety and more disorientation.

She was seen in follow-up sessions two weeks later, after taking Pamelor 30 mg nightly. She felt back to her old self. She was a forward-thinking, optimistic person.

The psychiatrist described her as "calm, in good control … not distressed or worried."

She called two weeks later and requested that the medication be increased. "Strange things in my head that come and go … like a twinge, a spark, as well as feeling very hot and flushed."

Pamelor was increased to 40 mg and an additional 10 mg as needed. When seen two weeks later, she was on the 50 mg but still occasionally feeling shaky, trembly inside, or extremely hot. For the most part, she felt well, hopeful, and energetic. She was having fun. Over the next six months, not encountering the previous severe symptoms, she requested the Nortriptyline be tapered and discontinued. But then there was a recrudescence.

"I'm on a roller coaster against my will. I can feel my body hardening. It's like screaming people are running through my body. This thing keeps rearing its ugly head. I don't even know who I am." She began sobbing. "I can't accomplish anything."

She was started on 50 mg of Zoloft (sertraline). After two and a half months, she said, "I've been much better generally. I can cope. There isn't this underlying feeling."

The patient appeared much more relaxed and was able to smile pleasantly. She requested an increase in the Zoloft to 75 mg so she could be totally without symptoms.

Several months later, she said, "It feels so good to me after so long—this magic that is coming out of nowhere."

The Zoloft 75 mg was continued. About four months later, she transitioned from Zoloft to Prozac (Fluoxetine) 20 mg. "I think it's a better medication for me." She noted feeling more rested, more even, and more focused, but the symptoms intruded. She began to feel crazed, anxious, tense, and toxic. She felt better after an increase to 30 mg.

At that juncture, she made an appointment for an evaluation with this writer. She was a very pleasant, attractive, soft-spoken, articulate, and intelligent young woman. She felt her previous psychiatrist was not helping her. She had been having appointments with him every other month. "He's so cold, and here I am desperately needing help. He's not accessible to me."

Her mother described here as a very carefree, cheerful child. On the day of the initial interview, she said, "I feel good."

She had no symptomatic complaints. She described her symptoms, anxiety attacks, and disorientation. "I don't even talk. I feel disoriented and crazy. I feel it's hopeless because it happens again. It's almost physical. My physical body changes. My skin crawls; it's not like any other physical sensation. I feel sick in my body, like just before I throw up. I just can't think. I can't put logical thoughts together. I feel disoriented, not of this world, like I don't belong here. I won't come out of it."

When she had symptoms, she was unable to conceptualize the positives in her life.

At the time of our initial interview, she was continuing with a therapist. In the first interview, she was composed, fairly relaxed, and affable, but the threat of her hideously severe, painful symptoms was lingering in the background.

At our next appointment, two weeks later, she reported another episode and then felt mediocre. The day before the appointment, she felt exceptionally well, clearheaded, and crisp. "My skin tone changes. I had food cravings, sugary things and caffeine, but the cravings were not present in the deepest phase."

She was reassured that she was not crazy, that she does come out of the symptoms, and that she wouldn't lose her son. She reassured herself about parenting. "I'll do it right. This is robbing me of my entire life, and I'll end up crazy in a padded cell."

Her Prozac was increased to 30 mg, and lithium was mentioned as a second medication. The risks and benefits were reviewed, and half a tablet was started about one month after the initial evaluation. For a period, she was feeling pretty well and clearheaded. She was able to function and was not having headaches. The instructions for the lithium was to increase by half a tablet every four days to a total of two tablets (600 mg). This dosage of lithium is at the lowest generally used dosage, which can range up to 1800 mg a day.

She did describe a brief period of aggression, little explosive moments. "I rubbed an egg on the wall; it wasn't in my nature to do this. As the lithium was slowly being increased, I was feeling sick to my stomach."

The lithium was discontinued for the time being, but she complained feeling angry and aggressive and in a funk. She reported a notable feeling of depression. "It's starting to escalate." It was punctuated by hyperalertness and aggression. The Prozac was reduced to 20 mg, and it was elected to try combination therapy. It was a combination of two antidepressants of different classes: Prozac, an SSRI, and Tofranil (imipramine), a tricyclic antidepressant. A very small dose, 10 mg, was increased to 20 mg and added to the Prozac.

Over the next two weeks, she described some really good days. "I'm pretty good."

At the end of May, her sleep became very disrupted. "I'm struggling to keep my eyes open."

We decided to hold the course with the Prozac 30 mg and Tofranil 20 mg. By the second week of June, she was more upbeat. "Actually, all in all, I'm better, some side effects."

She had just one day of mild depression. Laboratory tests were ordered to measure blood levels of Tofranil and thyroid-stimulating hormone (TSH).

On June 11, she described another terrible period. "I'm not coping, side effects, hard time holding on. I try so hard to bear it. I was trying to distract myself, but when I get like this, I can't think. I couldn't stay in the car or get out of it. I feel I'm on the edge. I feel crazy. I cannot think. I can't talk. It's so strange, I've had no relief in five days. It's like the other side of reality, like teetering." She was also complaining of somatic symptoms. "I'm shaky, sick to my stomach, it's constant for three days, my heart is racing."

She sounded in such distress, the option of hospitalization was introduced. It was reviewed with her the option of starting Risperdal (risperidone), a so-called second-generation antipsychotic medication that is also used as an adjunctive treatment for unipolar major depression and bipolar spectrum disorder. Risperdal was prescribed at a very low dosage: .5 mg. She did not start the Risperdal because she felt the Tofranil was causing her to be shaky. It was reduced from 20 mg to 10 mg.

She took the .5 mg Risperdal next. It was a mixed picture. The shaking was better. She declared she was feeling the best she had, but she also developed a rush in her abdomen, a swollen tongue, constipation, and very bizarre dreams. "My body isn't working right."

The Risperdal was stopped. Three alternative options were reviewed, a brief trial of Pamelor (nortriptyline), an alternative to Tofranil was added to the Prozac 20 mg, substituting the antianxiety Xanax (alprazolam) for Ativan (lorazepam), or considering a mood-stabilizer, Neurontin (gabapentin), which also has antianxiety properties.

She continued to feel poorly enough that she was considering hospitalization. By mid-July she had been able to tolerate Buspar (buspirone) a long-acting antianxiety agent, and 5 mg TID was added to the Prozac 20 mg.

"Things had improved enough that I haven't had to call. I'm feeling relatively well. At the end of July, I felt the toxic feeling" which was similar to when she was on Risperdal. She reduced the Buspar from one tablet three times daily to just one a day and started feeling "reasonably good."

We elected to raise the Buspar back up to three times daily. She again felt toxic but not as sick as last time.

In August, she decided the Prozac had not been helpful and discontinued it, but she began feeling more depressed. We elected to start Effexor (venlafaxine), which is classified as an SNRI (serotonin-noradrenaline reuptake inhibitor). She remained on Buspar 5 mg three times daily. It takes weeks to build up a new antidepressant, so she was feeling deeply depressed. "I feel I'm losing my mind."

The Effexor XR was started with one 37.5 mg tablet and very gradually, over six weeks, was raised to 225 mg, hoping to reach a treatment dosage. She had episodic symptoms: severe fatigue, feeling edgy, interrupted sleep, a painful, sick feeling high underneath her diaphragm, and constipation.

At the beginning of November, while on both Effexor 225 mg and Buspar 5 mg three times/daily, she felt she had a breakthrough. For three days, she hadn't needed the Ativan. In terms of medication, it was the best in three years. She reported sleeping deeply. She had a greater capacity to do things and felt in more control of her schedule. She did note, however, a sense of urgency. "I'm relentless about getting things done." This appeared to be evidence of hyperarousal.

In December, she was definitely better. She then experienced a bad patch: "Fighting low energy in addition to feeling hot, particularly at night, generally, I'm warmer all the time."

At the end of December, she reported feeling well, "pretty good." In early February, lab tests ordered by her family physician showed low platelets and white blood cells. A hematologist assured the undersigned her medications weren't the cause. It turned out to be a virus, and her lab results began to improve.

In early March, after attending a book club, she had terrible anxiety. "Shock running through my head, thoughts racing around, no way I could sleep, I was up all night."

Her Effexor was increased from 225 mg to 300 mg.

Toward the end of March, her white count had gone down more. Diagnostic tests, bone marrow biopsy, and CAT scan were scheduled. Her mood, however, was stable. Through April, she felt "generally it's a much better place." Her white count was improving. A Hamilton Depression Rating Scale score was 9, very close to full remission (≤7).

In early May, she became aware of feeling flat. "I'm not enjoying the usual pleasurable things. The Effexor was reduced back to 225 mg from 300 mg. Going down on the Effexor was a good thing but she hit a couple of days that were backsliding. She was having intense disturbing dreams.

Augmenting with Seroquel (quetiapine) was discussed. It is a second-generation antipsychotic, but it has other uses besides treating psychosis. It is also used as a mood stabilizer in bipolar spectrum mood disorders and as an augmentation for antidepressants in unipolar major depression. She was started on a low dose, 25 mg, at night. She reported feeling disconnected, fuzzy, and light-headed. "My eyes were really red, a big red blotch, it's not for me."

Toward the end of May, things were more positive again. "I'm doing acceptably well. It's acceptable right now, better than in the last four years, the blips are manageable." She felt she was able to get on with living her life.

At the end of June, she noted agitation, poor memory, and low energy. It was elected to increase Effexor back up to 300 mg during the premenstrual period and then reduce back to 225 mg. For the rest of August and September, her symptoms were generally milder.

At the end of December, her husband said, "She did really good over the past seven to eight months but is now worse."

She felt distraught and desperate that it would not go away. She again had the toxic feeling. The Effexor had been increased by 37.5 mg to 262.5 mg, but this was accompanied by severe fatigue and being in a fog. There were severe headaches. These were relieved when the Effexor was reduced back to 225 mg. Consideration was given to starting a mood stabilizer, Lamictal (lamotrigine). She was prescribed to start 25 mg at night. Her husband reported he noticed a difference, but she did not tolerate it.

In this interval her family physician made a diagnosis of Epstein-Barr virus, with a titer of 170, which he felt she had a long time, which was the cause of her depression. Her symptoms became worse. "I felt crazy … really bad … I couldn't think."

It took her a week to recover from the episode. By mid-January, she felt more stable. It was decided to add a small dose of Pamelor (nortriptyline) to the Effexor and then to cross-taper them by slowly lowering the Effexor while slowly raising the nortriptyline, but as we attempted this, she developed horrible withdrawal headaches. At the end of March, she reported, "I've been generally reasonably well." The Effexor helped prevent downs. She had returned to taking one Lamictal tablet, which made her feel a little more like herself, gentle, not just unwell, but well.

In May, her husband described her situation. "She's not feeling well enough … she's very uneven. She had two very severe anxiety attacks. Two Lorazepams only gave temporary relief. She had to take three. In addition, a number of days of depression … suicidal. Our objective is to have Sarah feeling the best."

A range of options was reviewed. She had positive feelings about Zoloft (sertraline) but also commented, "If I miss a day of Effexor or if you taper me off, I'd have to be hospitalized."

She felt desperate for relief, but she denied suicidal plans. "I love my life." Another trial of lithium was considered because of the history of bipolar illness in her family. She was started on a very low dose of a liquid form of lithium, 1 cc. At the end of June, she wasn't symptomatic on 150 mg of lithium.

"Feeling myself, I haven't in the past five years."

Her Hamilton Depression Rating Scale score was 3, well below the seven or less that indicates complete remission.

On August 1, her husband reported that she had stopped the lithium. "It wasn't doing anything." She was concerned that lithium brings down mania and could bring her down.

"Yesterday and the day before, two horrible days, crying uncontrollably, just bad. I was concerned the monster was rearing its head again … scared to death, what will happen … I don't want to leave my son. I feel my departure is imminent. I feel something will happen; it's that incredible feeling of doom."

She had suicidal thoughts. "To the depths of my soul, it's a drama, not that I'm going to do it. Worst episode I've ever had, four days so bad, horrible, taking sleeping pills, really unbearable, so extreme."

I became very ill in October, and Sarah sent a letter of sympathy and concern to my secretary.

This intelligent, pleasant, conscientious woman suffered agonies from a roller coaster of multiple, perplexing symptoms occurring almost unpredictably. Can anybody reading her case believe she could have stopped the symptoms by just deciding to do so?

Would anybody voluntarily subject themselves to the magnitude of ill-being, distress, helplessness, and pain characterizing her life? Yet she was a normal person. She would be perfectly pleasant company at a sophisticated dinner party. Was she mentally ill? No. Why add more pain? The pain of being labeled mental, as an additional burden of stigmatization, added to her severe symptoms.

In retrospect, given advances in psychiatric understanding of bipolar spectrum mood disorders, there might have been a more pronounced effort to utilize mood stabilizers and not antidepressants from the start of therapy. This illustrates the importance of expertise, experience, and advances in diagnostic knowledge.

Three Professors

Prof. V became my patient fifteen years before this writing. A very pleasant, self-spoken man, he held a position at an area university teaching physics. He had been on an old-style antidepressant, imipramine (Tofranil), a tricyclic, for several years, which had been switched to sertraline (Zoloft), which had no benefit, and then nortriptyline (Pamelor).

His most recent psychiatrist prescribed Serzone (another type of antidepressant), which made him very panicky. Finally, his primary care physician added fluoxetine (Prozac). In spite of this, his mood episodes were having a serious impact on his marriage. "She's had it with my depression. She says it's a roller coaster."

Through much of this period, he had continued in psychotherapy in addition to pharmacology. Diagnostic assessment indicated his severe, recurrent mood episodes could well be an expression of bipolar disorder. This he found a very upsetting notion; to him, manic-depressives were seriously mentally ill. He wanted no part of this assertion.

It was explained there are variants of illness subsumed under the bipolar category, and his particular illness was not strictly manic depression, but a bipolar II illness in which recurrent clinical depressions are the central feature and not severe manias.

It was also explained antidepressants alone should not be the mainstay of treatment, but only an occasional addition to mood stabilizers, which include anticonvulsants (the same medications prescribed for neurological disorders) and/or lithium.

Again, he found lithium as a treatment option upsetting. It had a connotation to him of being used for the severely mentally ill: "Wild-looking, unkempt, ragged, obviously crazy individuals came to my mind."

He responded to a discussion with examples of many intelligent, successful, creative individuals who have been immensely helped by lithium. Indeed, it is kind of an aphrodisiac for brain cells, embellishing their connections (synapses) and preventing apoptosis, the suicide machinery of the neuron, which kills them.

The major mood illnesses are very difficult illnesses. Under treatment over the years, Professor V has had periods of clinical depression, though the overall level of symptoms has been far less intense and shorter in duration. His academic work has been successful. He has continued his athletic activities as a long-distance and marathon runner while continuing to take prescribed lithium. His long-term maintenance medications also include lamotrigine (Lamictal), an anticonvulsant that may have preferential benefit for bipolar spectrum illnesses.

An Update on Professor V

About a year and a half prior to completion of this report, his father died. He began to notice mild depression. A Hamilton Depression Rating Scale score of 11½ (above the 7 that indicates full remission) was consistent with this. He also started to have more than the usual side effects of tremors and feeling unsteady.

His mild depression persisted. Ultimately, because of the persistence of tremors in spite of an antidote (propranolol, a beta-blocker), it was decided to taper and stop lithium.

Unfortunately, soon after his Hamilton Rating Scale Score increased to 17½, indicating a worsening of his clinical depression. Several medication switches and adjustments were attempted.

He was having cardiovascular symptoms, but the tests and labs were normal. There were irregularities of blood pressure for which he consulted his internist. He also underwent neurological evaluation, including an MRI of the brain and EMGs (for nerve symptoms like burning and tingling).

About four months later, after working with Provigil (modafinil), an energizing medication, he was having a little less difficulty getting up in the morning and forcing himself to get ready for work. He had been very worried he could not mobilize sufficiently to make it to work).

At the beginning of the summer, we reviewed replacing lithium with Abilify (apiprazole), a drug used for three indications, in higher dosage for more severe disorders such as schizophrenia, and in more moderate dosage as a mood-stabilizer for bipolar spectrum illnesses or as an adjunct to antidepressants in severe unipolar major depression.

The dosage was titrated up by increments of 2 mg to 6 mg (it can be raised as high as 30 mg). Immediately prior to starting Abilify, he described his general situation as a "tangle." He felt he was slipping down, feeling especially discouraged and depressed.

A month later, he observed that seven to ten days after the Abilify started, he began to feel much improved. "Doing very well …

amazing … my anxiety is way down." His difficulty in getting going in the morning was gone. His sleep was enormously improved. He felt very motivated. "Best I've felt in a long time." In the opinion of this author, Professor V, a successful professor and pleasant man, is not mentally ill.

Professor G

Professor G originally was seen in consultation, having a playful glint in her eye and a matching sense of humor. A very attractive woman, she was socially very pleasant and at ease. Her major depressive illness, at first masked by alcohol dependence, was diagnosed ten years previously when she became abstinent. She had been started on an old-style antidepressant, Tofranil (imipramine), but symptoms had broken through.

Her therapist suggested she be reevaluated for clinical depression. For six months, she had increasing difficulties making decisions, had to struggle to motivate herself, and had strong urges to withdraw from routines and just sleep. Her outlook changed, and even activities she enjoyed seemed like a bit of a drag. She was unusually fatigued and tired.

About a year and a half later, she was not taking an antidepressant, but symptoms began to encroach on her quality of life: profound fatigue, uncharacteristic irritability, and more powerful cravings for sweets. She started fluoxetine (Prozac 10 mg). Over the next ten years, it became necessary to increase the dosage to 40 mg and then augment it with another type of antidepressant, Wellbutrin (bupropion), ultimately adjusted to 300 mg.

She misplaced her Wellbutrin prescription and described the early, more subtle symptoms of an incipient mood episode. "It's more difficult to keep a good attitude. I'm more easily overwhelmed. I think, *What's the point?* I feel things are useless."

Soon after the Wellbutrin was started, she felt a return to her usual self. This charming professor by then had spent hundreds of hours lecturing to thousands of students. She at no point should be labeled mentally ill.

Professor A

Professor A, a man in his late forties, came for his original consultation about twenty years before this writing. A tall, handsome man, he had an aspect of complete gentleness. Soft and well-spoken, he elaborated on a roster of symptoms that were undermining his well-being: severe headaches, chronic sinus infections, numbness, disorientation, hypersensitivity to light, inability to concentrate, impaired coordination, weakness, hearing difficulty, excessive skin flushing, fatigue, insomnia, heart palpitations, irritability, esophageal reflux, and difficulty swallowing.

An esophageal biopsy was planned to rule out cancer. About his overall situation, he felt embattled, sad, and despairing. "I'll ever get better, and I'll just drop off and go insane or collapse." He had had suicidal thoughts—but no actual plan.

Well, he did not drop off or go insane over the next two decades. He continued lecturing and teaching throughout that time. Ultimately, a particular antidepressant, Lexapro (escitalopram), was a source of symptomatic improvement. Although he dealt with a number of stresses over the years, he was always gracious in his manner, his presence contributing to a calm, pleasant ambience. It is a gross misrepresentation to label him mentally ill.

Three Gracious Women

Kate N had been my patient for fourteen years before this writing. Her depressive illness had started in third grade. "I've always had depression."

She had been on Zoloft for four years and came to our first appointment to renew her antidepressant therapy. She had a habit of compulsive counting repeatedly from 1–10, like a song in her head.

She was a soft-spoken young woman with light brown hair and

blue eyes. Clinical evaluation demonstrated severe major depression, the seventeen-item HAM-D score was 44, accompanied by extremes of depressed mood, guilt, a sense of emptiness about her life, disrupted concentration, irritability, autonomic signs of anxiety (palpitations, hyperventilation), panicky feeling, loss of appetite, and debilitating fatigue and exhaustion. Her quality of life was markedly degraded by her symptoms.

She was restarted on Zoloft (sertraline). One month later, her HAM-D had dropped to 16, and then in the next month to 3. Her mood was spontaneously cheerful, and her outlook was more positive and optimistic. She no longer felt emptiness, unreasonable guilt, severe anxiety, or fatigue. Her concentration was again sharply focused. It was quite a transformation.

Over the years, however, her depressive episodes were an expression of a type of bipolar disorder (type 2), in which severe so-called manic episodes don't occur. This revised diagnosis was made over time when she appeared to have a few days episodically of feeling better than her nondepressed, baseline mood, a bit more energetic, active, and optimistic.

Also, a history of subtly elevated moods was noted in her teens and early twenties. At times, she overconsumed alcohol and decided to become abstinent while attending a support group to facilitate this. She was transitioned to lithium and Zoloft.

For a considerable period, she felt quite well: ("My mood is fine, as smooth as silk." In 2009, she expressed a desire to finally stop smoking, and she was familiar with a medication, Chantix, which had the indication for smoking cessation. During this trial, she developed insomnia, increasing inner agitation, irritability, and dysphoria. Her HAM-D peaked at 36½.

An additional medication, an atypical neuroleptic, Seroquel (quetiapine), was added. Her HAM-D descended to 13. Even though the Seroquel seemed to help lower her symptoms, she was bothered by a side effect, and it was discontinued. She did feel much improved: "good … mentally on track … thinking correctly."

In May of 2013, she experienced some depressive symptoms (HAM-D 18½), and the Lamictal was increased from 150 mg to 200 mg. She noted, "I'm definitely improved, more focused." The HAM-D was back to normal (5).

This personable, intelligent, competent woman does indeed have a significant brain dysregulation for which she assumed full responsibility to seek out treatment. It sticks in my craw to stigmatize her by labeling her mentally ill.

***

Alice became my patient eight years prior to this writing, at the age of twenty-two years. A charming, pleasant young woman, her depressive episodes had started when she was seventeen in college. She lost friends, withdrew, and slept all the time. She noted an underlying sadness, anxiety about schoolwork, and feeling rejected socially.

She had been to England and had a romantic relationship with a young man. He dumped her, but she still loved England and wanted to return. She felt English children were so cute and wanted to teach there.

At the time of the initial visit, the Hamilton Depression Rating scale score was 54 on the seventeen-item scale. She was struggling. At times, she felt so alone and hopeless. "I'd have suicidal thoughts, but I'd never do it."

She developed extreme tension, distress, and anxiety because of a fear she might have a horrible disease. She spent many miserable hours doing research to try to rule out distressing possibilities. On Lexapro (Escitalopram) at a dosage of 20 mg, she noted things were improving. She was socially more active. "I met a nice guy."

She was able to refrain from repeatedly palpating her lymph nodes. "I didn't feel people were coming at me and recovered from my crying spells." Her HAM-D score decreased to 15.

She was making plans to return to England to teach and continued to improve. "I'm absolutely fine … no mood swings … trazodone helps me sleep."

Prior to her departure to England, I prepared a clinical note to hand to her treating physician there. She spent a year there. About a year later, she developed another severe depressive episode with panic attacks. She became extremely preoccupied about having a serious disease and was spending hours examining herself in the mirror. "It's taken away my life."

Her Lexapro was increased from 20 to 30 mg, and was augmented with Wellbutrin (bupropion), eventually 300 mg. And Klonopin (clonazepam) specifically for panic attacks. Her HAM-D score, which had reached 47½ (consistent with severe major depression) slowly came down to 18, and then to 8.

"I feel very good … much better."

This charming, pleasant young woman had severe symptoms, but I refuse to think of her as being mentally ill.

***

Rebecca was a tall, blonde, soft-spoken young teacher. She became noticeably enthusiastic when she discussed her teaching duties. Over the years, even though she had at times profound inner doubts about her competence, her professionalism and genuine abilities led to ongoing recognition by her principals. She was favored for teaching gifted classes.

She managed to continue making her contribution to the education and well-being of her students every year—in spite of struggling with a severe recurrent mood illness.

Her depression started in the third grade. There was a family history of similar illness; her father had once been hospitalized, and two paternal relatives had committed suicide. She had been prescribed Effexor in the past, and since she felt it had helped her mood, it was prescribed.

A month later, she felt considerable improvement in her outlook and mood. For a two-year period, she felt reasonably well, but then she relapsed into a major depressive episode. Her HAM-D score spiked at 26½. Recurrent symptoms included severe insomnia, apathy, loss of capacity to retain interest and enjoyment in favored activities, uncontrolled worrying, and extreme fatigue.

This episode cleared up slowly. Three months later, the HAM-D score had returned to 7. Two years later, she experienced severe obsessive thoughts centered on the theme of professional failure accompanied by panic attacks and clinical depression.

She was being prescribed lithium and Lamotrigine. The dose of the latter was increased to 500 mg. About a year later, she again entered a bad phase. My moods are all over the place … it hasn't been this bad in years. I can't do anything right. I can't stop worrying. I can't relax … I can't stay in bed. Assessment week, I was so depressed and stressed out. I was yelling and screaming awful. Once I started taking Risperdal, I was feeling better."

At the end of the year it was decided to cross-taper from Risperdal to Abilify, a newer medication. Unfortunately, there were additional severe depressive episodes over the next several years, but she was able to continue teaching and have periods of improved mood and well-being.

Then she had a manic episode. "The impulses are so strong. I have rapid speech … I'm not sleeping … I'm saying inappropriate things."

The Young Mania Rating Scale Score was 25. The Abilify was increased. Over the next two years, she was chosen for select teaching positions and assignments.

It is distasteful and cruel to add to the emotional discomfort her illness has caused by labeling her as mentally ill.

Two Patients with Obsessive Compulsive Disorder

J became my patient twelve years before this writing. He had been laid off several months earlier, and his father died around that time of a stroke. He had nagging doubt that he could have done more to save his father. "I feel responsible … I could have done it differently … I should have been more proactive … The neurosurgeon saw him at six o'clock, but it was too late. If he had agreed to a breathing tube, would he still be alive?"

He had had symptoms of anxiety off and on for twenty years and had previously been prescribed Tofranil (imipramine), then Ludiomil (maprotiline), then Wellbutrin (bupropion) over the years, but had subsequently weaned himself off.

About a year later, he felt worse. His primary care doctor prescribed Paxil (paroxetine), but he stopped it due to sexual side effects. Subsequently, his symptoms became worse. "I feel the anxiety is overtaking my mind. I have no family, no job. I don't see a way forward."

In particular, two sets of symptoms were requiring more and more exertion and resulting in more and more fatigue. When laundering his clothes, he had to insert the individual items of clothes in a particular order and then keep repeating the sequence because he had to get it done in a specific way, then doubting he had done it correctly.

In addition, when leaving his house, he was overcome by a strong preoccupation that he had forgotten something very important, causing him to reenter the house to check it out. This unwelcome compulsion could keep him tied up for an unwarranted length of time.

The MINI International Neuro-Psychiatric Interview was administered. It was clearly positive for obsessive-compulsive disorder. The initial Hamilton Depression Rating Scale score was also significantly elevated at 25, with significant symptoms of excessive self-reproach, a sense of emptiness about his life, insomnia, particularly difficulty falling asleep, loss of interest in previously enjoyable activities, disrupted concentration, inner restlessness, unusual fatigue, and feelings of hopelessness.

He was started on Zoloft (sertraline) on a step-wise escalation, a dosage of up to 200 mg usually the highest dosage. Over a three-month period, the HAM-D score transitioned to 16, next 14, and then 6.

The Zoloft was helping the OCD, and he was able to leave the house without having to return to check. He summed up the symptomatic improvement. "This week, I feel pretty good, and I'm getting a few things done." In spite of the overall improvement, he felt a little blasé. The addition of Wellbutrin (bupropion) to the Zoloft alleviated it.

He had bereavement when his mother passed away—but not clinical depression. Over the ensuing decade, he continued his medication. The OCD was no more than a twinge. He does some consulting and monitors his own investing.

Bob is an intelligent, personable if shy man who should not be categorized as mentally ill.

***

OCD is an interesting illness. Whoever or whatever thought it up outdid themselves in creating curious phenomena. It is no walk in the park or gentle zephyr; it ties up the lives of those who are unfortunate enough to have the affliction. Underlying the symptoms are gross dysregulation of physical brain circuits not subject to voluntary control or will. In particular, serotonergic neurotransmission is problematically disruptive.

Beatrice was my patient for fifteen years prior to this writing. Her OCD symptoms became noticeable in childhood when she had to make sure her blankets and sheets were absolutely smooth. In her early adult years, in spite of tenacious determination to put a stop to her symptoms, she simply was powerless to do so. Hours each day were consumed by useless repetitive activities, staying up all night counting and recounting silverware, or making sure the fringes on her carpets were absolutely straight. She was unable to hold a job, experiencing paralyzing repetitive behaviors in that circumstance, although she felt a desire to be employed. She had become increasingly isolated and lonely. Symptoms became so oppressive in her early twenties that hospitalization was necessary.

Throughout this period, she had been on a number of medications, an old tricyclic medication, Prozac, Anafranil, lithium, an MAO-inhibiter (Nardil), clonidine, and Tegretol. She had participated in behavior therapy. In the hospital, she had a course of 15 ECT, which alleviated clinical depression but not the OCD. Subsequently, she also had trials of Eldepryl (an MAOI-inhibitor), phenylalanine, and fluoxetine. She had additional behavior therapy. In spite of these interventions, she remained incapacitated.

When I met her at our first appointment, one could not discern by her manner or presentation that she was so persecuted by the OCD illness. She was very pleasant, soft-spoken, attractive, well-attired, and had considerable charm. We decided to arrange a special consultation with an OCD doctor. He recommended increasing her daily dose of Zoloft up to double the standard highest dose—400 mg—and a trial of a glutamate-modulating agent. He recommended discontinuing the Abilify in spite of the initial dramatic but transitory improvement in the OCD.

Subsequently, she had a severe major depressive episode. There was a pervasive sense of emptiness about her life, insomnia, inability to enjoy or obtain pleasure from previously rewarding activities, severe inner agitation and restlessness, marked irritability, cardiovascular symptoms of palpitations, and de-enervating fatigue. The HAM-D score was 29. Three weeks later, after restoration of the Abilify at a lower dosage, she was much improved. The HAM-D score was reduced to 8. As our next pharmacological step, the Zoloft was slowly being increased to 325 mg. Her mood has remained satisfactory. She has noted that she can complete cleaning a room in less time and with less interference from checking behavior.

Our pharmacological objective is to continue, slowly increasing the Zoloft to 400 mg and then considering a glutamatergic agent. In spite of her symptomatic sufferings, her good-naturedness and warmth are apparent. She combines a gracious countenance with determination and forbearance. The stereotypes evoked by labeling her mentally ill are totally inappropriate and should not be inflicted on her—or on anyone else.

Two Clergymen

Father B was a priest and a social worker A gentle, kindly, very warm, and intelligent man, he had recently been struggling with health issues: a severe case of shingles, especially causing pain in his face, and recurrent, severe sinusitis, which required sinus surgery. The facial shingles was starting to improve, but he remained very tired. "I have no energy … I'm not sleeping."

He had been prescribed Paxil (paroxetine) 20 mg over the past several months, but it wasn't helping. "It's a burden to talk to people … I've just lost my interest, and it's hard to focus and read."

He was finding it more difficult to maintain his active schedule. The Hamilton Depression Rating Scale score was 28, consistent with severe major clinical depression. Significant symptoms were a severe sense of emptiness, initial insomnia, loss of enjoyment and interest, interference with concentration, loss of interest in food and eating, lack of energy and chronic tiredness, and feeling unusually self-reproachful. The initial pharmacological intervention was a prescription of Lexapro (escitalopram) after the Paxil was tapered and discontinued. The Lexapro dosage was increased to 20 mg from 10 mg.

Three weeks later, his HAM-D score was reduced to 12 (considered a response which is defined as a 50 percent reduction in the original HAM-D value). "Overall this week, I can feel the improvement, and I'm getting back the energy."

By the end of year, however, he wasn't feeling as well. The neuropathic facial pain was still very bothersome, and the pain triggered depression. It was decided to taper Lexapro and replace it with Cymbalta (duloxetine) when a new HAM-D assessment scored 24, a significant worsening from the previous score of 12. The Cymbalta was stabilized at a dosage of 30 mg twice a day.

Over the next several weeks, he reported, "It's effective … it seems to be working. I'm able to function." His mood was much improved. His enthusiasm for his clerical and therapeutic responsibilities returned. He was increasing his client load in practice and his hobbies and leisure interests. He was gardening and tending to the trees on the property where he resides.

The Cymbalta was doing its job.

A robust octogenarian, he continues his very active schedule. Father B—a source of sustenance and support to thousands of parishioners and clients for over four decades—is insultingly mischaracterized by being labeled mentally ill.

***

When Father W came in for his initial evaluation, he was fifty-seven. He had been very active in his clerical duties and, after a period of cardiovascular illnesses, he acknowledged that he had been working more than he should have. He found it increasingly difficult to make decisions and had a lot of trouble thinking.

His sister said, "I think he did too much—the extra night work he's doing—and he hasn't taken a day off in two months."

Father W was apprehensive about keeping up with his schedule and thought he might lose his position. His Hamilton Depression Rating score was 42 (demonstrating severe major depression) with predominant symptoms, severe anhedonia, extreme interruption of concentration and inner agitation, severe physical anxiety and irritability accompanied by insomnia and great fatigue. Effexor XR (venlaxine) 37.5 mg tablets were initiated, increasing the dosage to four tablets (150 mg total dosage) over approximately two weeks. In about four weeks, he acknowledged feeling and sleeping much better.

The Effexor dosage was stabilized at 75 mg twice daily. He noted he was more like his old self. He transitioned to a dysphoric mood. His sleep was again interrupted, and he was increasingly agitated and restless. It was difficult to sit down. His thinking seemed confused, his concentration was erratic, and he couldn't think in an ordered fashion about his many tasks and responsibilities. "I don't feel in control."

He became fearful that he would lose his position at his parish. It was noted in his history, about twenty years earlier, he had experienced a period of several months in which he felt immobilized and was unable to function as usual. This was interpreted as a possible mixed mood episode, possibly a sign of atypical bipolar disorder, although there was no typical history of manic symptoms. Then he learned he was being relieved of his current official duties and would transition into phased retirement. His sister was concerned. "He loves what he's doing, but he seemed to adapt gracefully enough to his retirement."

He said, "Symptomatically, I feel better … no racing of my thoughts … the confusion is getting better."

In addition to his mood illness, he had advanced cardiovascular disease and was being monitored at Columbia Presbyterian Medical Center for a possible heart transplant.

About a year and a half after the initiation of treatment, he again experienced mood symptoms. "If I could get my thinking under control." The HAM-D score was again elevated to 17½ (though much lower than the original score of 42 at the time of his initial evaluation). An initial dosage of another medication used to treat bipolar illness, Zyprexa (olanzapine) 2.5 mg, was added. (The Effexor had been previously stopped.)

In about five weeks, the HAM-D score had dropped to 4. About a year later, he seemed to be developing hints of side effects to Zyprexa. Slowly, another mood stabilizer-anticonvulsant was added, and then Zyprexa was withdrawn.

Several months later, his sister reported that Father W had seemed unusually activated for a period, making inappropriate advances in public places. When evaluated, it was learned he had been missing his medication doses. This episode was self-limited. Until his death, about a year and a half later after a heart attack, he remained eager to lend a hand to parishes, especially around Easter. His sister remarked that he was held in high esteem in church circles.

In my opinion, Father W was not mentally ill.

Two Attorneys

Mr. L became my patient fifteen years prior to this writing. He noted that his wife had pointed out to him that he didn't smile and didn't seem to enjoy his life at all. Over the past two and a half years, he had a more negative outlook, a sadness prevailing in his mood. He described himself as lacking oomph, feeling lethargic. He had seen a GP about these complaints and was told to return in five months.

He had a private law practice that it was not as lucrative as it could have been because he spent a lot of time with clients who were hurting … troubled people. He also derived satisfaction from pro bono work for charities.

His HAM-D score was 26, consistent with moderately severe major depression. Significant symptoms included insomnia, inability to really enjoy activities (anhedonia), deficient interest levels, restlessness, an inner agitation, excessive worrying and ruminations, low energy, fatigue, and loss of libido. He was prescribed Celexa (citalopram).

A month later, the HAM-D score was significantly reduced to 12. By definition, this is consistent with a good response to the citalopram (HAM-D reduction by 50 percent) but not yet a complete remission (HAM-D of 7 or less). He had been able to have an extraordinarily wonderful time at his twenty-fifth class reunion over the recent weekend, a promising note.

Approximately two months after starting Celexa, the HAM-D was reduced to remission range (5). “For the most part, I feel fine … relatively calm … different than last time … coping … getting more sleep … cooking along. I’m less grumpy at home.”

About six months later, however, he said, “I’m kind of tired. I don’t have a lot of oomph … a wet noodle.” His HAM-D score was significantly elevated to 21. A second antidepressant, Wellbutrin (bupropion) was added to the Celexa (combination therapy). Three weeks later, the score had lowered to 8. He had a feeling of well-being.

Mr. C, an attorney who extended himself to clients who could ill afford the usual legal fees, should not be categorized as mentally ill.

***

Mrs. P was a practicing attorney. She complained of being increasingly anxious and stressed due to cumulative work pressures.

She felt she was not getting things done. She was particularly concerned about the impact of the stress on her blood pressure. "I'm on so many blood pressure medications." Her energy was in short supply, and she complained of always being backlogged. Prominent symptoms included a seriously altered mood, severe self-reproach, insomnia, impaired concentration, inner restlessness and agitation, constant ruminations, irritability, fatigue, and severely reduced energy levels. The Hamilton Depression scale score was 29½, consistent with severe major depression. Celexa (citalopram) was prescribed.

Three weeks later, the HAM-D had fallen to 17, and by six weeks, to 7. She reported that she was a lot better. "I cope with everything a lot better, and I'm more energetic too."

She still felt fatigued. Wellbutrin (bupropion), a second antidepressant that can improve energy and fatigue but does little for anxiety, was added to the citalopram (combination therapy).

"Wellbutrin helps me make it through the day … I'm more awake … I'm getting a lot more done."

Several months later, however, she said, "I felt anxiety coming back." The escitalopram and Wellbutrin dosages were raised. "I'm on the edge of anxiety … but it's manageable."

A couple of years later, she was able to retire. She had a long-standing interest in improving educational opportunities for poor children, and now she could devote much more time to her projects for them. She was instrumental in founding a nutrition center and dental clinic in a rural area. Another unrelated endeavor she had great enthusiasm for was teaching art to women who otherwise had no opportunities to experience advanced cultural activities.

In my opinion, this creative and compassionate person should not be classified as or thought of as being mentally ill.

GLOSSARY

therapy psychiatrist. Conducts prolonged forty-five-minute psychotherapy with each patient, generally weekly with a duration of several years. Not a student of the brain, its structure, or processes.

amygdala. A set of neurons linked to fear and pleasure responses.

anhedonia. Inability to experience pleasure or joy.

antipsychotic. Class of medications used to treat psychotic illnesses, but also many other conditions.

bipolar affective disorder. Mood illness characterized by clinical depression, but also hypomania or mania.

brain psychiatrist. Prioritizes studying the brain in detail and basing pharmacological treatments on this in-depth understanding. Does not do forty-five-minute weekly psychotherapy.

cingulate gyrus. Important part of the limbic system, which regulates emotion and pain.

cognitive deficits. Impairment in mental processes like learning and memory.

cortex. Brain's outer layer, which contains neurons.

cortisol. An adrenal hormone that modulates stress responses.

cytokines. Small protein molecules active in the immune and inflammatory processes in the brain.

dexamethasone depression test. Assesses adrenal functions and may be abnormal in MDD.

ECT (electroconvulsive therapy). Triggering a mild seizure that relieves severe depression. A medical procedure.

glutamate. An amino acid neurotransmitter, generally having excitatory effects on neurons.

gray matter. The brain substance containing neurons.

hippocampus. The part of the brain involved in memory formation and memory storing. It is part of the limbic system.

insula. A part of the cerebral cortex associated with visceral function.

limbic system. Set of brain structures buried under the cortex and involved in emotions and motivations.

lithium. lithium salts, used in the treatment of mood disorders.

major depressive disorder. The most common form of severe (clinical) mood illness.

mental health care system. The so-called alternate health care system, in which the mentally ill receive services. It isolates itself from the general medical system.

methylphenidate. A medication used to treat ADHD, and as an augmentation (added to other medications) in other psychiatric disorders.

mood stabilizer. Also known as anticonvulsants, used to treat epilepsy and bipolar disorders.

monotherapy. The utilization of only one psychotropic medication at a time.

MRI imaging. A medical imaging technique used to image the anatomy and physiological process of diseases.

multiple sclerosis. A disease that attacks the insulating covers (myelin) of nerves, affecting the brain and spinal cord.

myelinated. Of a nerve, having a myelin sheath.

poststroke depression. A severe mood episode following a cerebral vascular accident.

psychopharmacology. The study of medications used to treat mental disorders. Complex field that requires continuous study to keep current with advances.

receptor. A structure that receives signals from outside a cell and transmits it to inside the cell.

receptor agonist. A substance activating a receptor.

serotonin. A monoamine neurotransmitter.

serotonin IA receptor. A subtype of serotonin receptor that binds serotonin.

temporal lobe epilepsy. A subtype of epilepsy, characterized by focal seizures, partial versus full-blown grand mal.

CHAPTER 3

The Treacherous Dichotomy

Psychiatry has divided all human illnesses into two broad categories: diseases of the physical body diagnosed and treated by physicians, and mental illnesses, in which deep mental conflicts result in symptoms and suffering. Physical diseases with simple physical causes do not require sophisticated therapies, as do mental illnesses, in which therapy psychiatrists, by virtue of specialized training in psychoanalytically oriented psychotherapy employ deft psychoanalytic interpretations in the course of long-term therapy, exposing and healing deep psychological scars. The physical diseases are predictably diagnosed and treated physically. The mental illnesses, however, require a separate system, the mental health care system, so the sophisticated psychotherapeutic techniques therapy psychiatrists utilize are not diluted by simplified notions there could be physical causes of mental illnesses.

The reality of human illness is that there is no separation between them into this archaic bifurcation. It is overridden, and the mental health care system is perpetuated. The therapy psychiatrist's mental patients receive little or no attention from physicians for their physical problems and vice versa.

The objective of any health care system should be the prevention of diseases, the early detection and treatment of them, or the reduction of symptoms and disabilities. The current dichotomous approach fails the test of prevention on all three levels because the synergies they would require are not possible when symptoms and suffering are so arbitrarily divided and conceptualized. The resulting cast of mind fosters a delusional belief in fictitious categories around which providers coalesce in isolation from each other.

Kate Scott, PhD, et al[5] investigated the association of sixteen mental disorders to ten physical illnesses. (They arbitrarily use the mental-physical dichotomy, but how could they know any better given therapy psychiatry's confirmed embracement of the dichotomy?) They used data from face-to-face household interviews of 47,609 individuals across seventeen countries between January 1, 2001, and December 31, 2011.

The mental disorders included depressive disorders, anxiety disorders, including panic disorder, post-traumatic stress disorder, bipolar disorder, social phobia and other phobias, among others. They physical conditions were heart disease, stroke, cancer, diabetes mellitus, hypertension, asthma, chronic lung disease, peptic ulcer, arthritis, chronic back or neck pain, chronic pain disorders. Mental disorders of all kinds were statistically associated with increases in a wide range of physical illnesses; the more severe the mental disorders, the greater incidence of physical illnesses. For example, a history of a depressive episodes was associated with increased odds of subsequent arthritis.

Significant associations ranged from 150 percent to 200 percent greater increases of the physical illnesses. In contrast to individuals not having mental illness, they conclude the deleterious effects of mental disorders on physical health accumulate over the life course, and the more severe the mental illnesses, the proportionally more severe the physical illnesses. They note the disappointing outcomes of treatment assessments, for example, of patients with heart disease and comorbid depression and vice versa. They recommend the mental-physical comorbidity be addressed by an earlier focus on the physical

---

[5] Association of Mental Disorders with Subsequent Chronic Physical Conditions World Mental Health Surveys from Seventeen Countries.

health of people with mental disorders. (Good luck with that ... what is asunder cannot simultaneously be an integrated whole.)

Andres M. Kanner, a distinguished neurologist, MD, has a particular interest in the relationship between neurological illnesses and mood disorders, and has published on the topic.[6] His keen interest is in direct contrast to most neurologists; there is such apathy about paying attention to comorbid depressive disorders in neurologic conditions that there is no good data on their treatment. This is not a surprise since neurologists and psychiatrists do not have a common language. Psychiatrists operate in their own isolated, mental health care system.

Since he is making his comments in a neurological journal, he is evidently interested in enlightening neurologists. He notes that mood disorders are associated with neurotransmitter and neuroendocrine disturbances, which result in structural and functional changes in the brain. That probably explains why the course of neurological conditions in patients with depression result in worse outcomes than patients without depression. Neurological and mood disorders share common pathogenic mechanisms. For example, there is decreased binding of serotonin[7] to the serotonin IA receptors in the hippocampus, insula, amygdala, cingulate gyrus, and raphe nuclei in depression and temporal lobe epilepsy.

Depression is associated with low-platelet serotonin, which increases clotting and increased secretion of cytokines, which may be associated with vasculitic processes, both of which may increase the risk of strokes. One of the neurotransmitters implicated in seizures, glutamate, is also present in high levels in the cortex of patients with depression. People with neurological disorders, stroke, epilepsy,

---

[6] Kanner AM, Schachter [SIC], Barry JJ, et al. Depression and epilepsy and epidemiologic and neurobiological perspectives that may explain their high comorbid occurrence. *Epilepsy Behav.* 2012; 24(2): 156–168. Kublubaev MA, Hackett Emily. Part II: predictors of depression after stroke and impact of depression on stroke outcome: an updated systemic review of observational studies. *Int. J. Stroke.* 2014; 9 (8): 1026

[7] Refer to glossary for definitions.

migraine, and Parkinson's disease have a 33 percent higher probability of developing MDD than the general population. Between 27 and 54 percent of patients with multiple sclerosis also develop MDD. In other words, there is a bidirectional relationship that people with major neurological illnesses are more likely to develop MDD and vice versa.

He discusses in more detail the effect of depression on patients who have had a stroke. In contrast to similar patients without depression, the dually affected individuals have a greater degree of cognitive deficits and impairment. Two years after a stroke, they have poorer recovery of basic living skills (activities of daily living), and their mortality risk is 50 percent higher than those without poststroke depression. It is quite likely that the gulf separating neurologist from having services of qualified brain psychiatrists, there being too few, account for these morbid outcomes. Most neurologists don't know a therapy from a brain psychiatrist anyway, and the therapy psychiatrists are holed up in their isolated mental health care system. How could the stroke victims or their families ever comprehend this conundrum? The patients with poststroke depression become more ill than necessary and die, and their families suffer and grieve.

Multiple sclerosis, unlike stroke, affects young and middle-aged people. Dr. Anthony Feinstein, PhD, of Sunnybrook Health Sciences Center in Toronto, has stated that when you've got a disease without a cure affecting young and middle-aged people, good symptom management becomes important.[8] He states available therapies for neuropsychiatric disorders (at least Dr. Feinstein does not call them mental disorders) can improve quality of life for patients with MS, so the diagnosis should not be missed.

Guess what? The psychiatrists who should be responsible for educating neurologists about the physical basis for neuropsychiatric disorders are for the most part off in their own mental health care system cocoons, from which they issue forth incisive psychodynamic

---

[8] Neuropsychiatric Disorders in MS are Common and Treatable; *Neurology Reviews*, 2015 2, 3(1):17.

interpretations to expose and heal the deep conflicts of their analysands (therapy patients).

Dr. Feinstein observes patients with multiple sclerosis have a 50 percent likelihood of developing comorbid depression. He notes some of the prominent symptoms—changes in appetite, insomnia, fatigue, and inability to concentrate—are hallmarks of depression. (He does not mention anhedonia, the symptom robbing a severely depressed person's ability to experience any enjoyment, interest, pleasure, or hope), perhaps the most tormenting symptom, but he means well. He outlines a diagnostic and therapeutic protocol for neurologists. First, not to miss the diagnosis, which can be detected using appropriate self-report questionnaires and a particular laboratory examination, the dexamethasone suppression test, in which the patient's cortisol level remains high after a single dose of dexamethasone. He outlines a series of treatment steps for neurologists: first monotherapy with an SSRI. If that fails, use of an SNRI like bupropion or mirtazapine (neither of which causes sexual side effects). If the patient fails to respond to monotherapy, combination therapy can be appropriate, which in addition to a second antidepressant, could include an antidepressant plus methylphenidate or lithium carbonate. He continues, if these approaches have not succeeded, electroconvulsive therapy could. He states ECT is a safe treatment in multiple sclerosis, provided the neurologist rules out the active phase of MS by ordering a gadolinium-enhanced MRI before proceeding to ECT. He concludes that ECT is quite safe, and the response rate is excellent.

Dr. Feinstein observes bipolar affective disorder is twice as common among individuals with MS as it is in the general population. He advises neurologists to consult the psychiatric literature for details of treatment (they better, as therapy psychiatrists just prescribe pills rather than practicing sophisticated psychopharmacology). Dr. Feinstein continues, "Patients respond well to mood-stabilizing medication such as lithium or valproic acid." He observes, "If your patient is psychotic, occasionally you have to introduce an antipsychotic agent as well."

Camera, camera on the wall … how many neurologists actually follow Dr. Feinstein's protocol? Probably very few, as it is actually much more trying in the details than the outline implies. His protocol is actually part of the practice of sophisticated psychopharmacology, which therapy psychiatrists don't practice either. They, like neurologists, don't generally research the psychiatric (misnomer—it should be psychopharmacologic) literature.

An interesting medical tidbit from a study published in *Molecular Psychiatry* was summarized in *Psychiatry Advisor* on December 28, 2015. Alan R. Prossin, MD, from the University of Texas Health Science Center at Houston and colleagues hypothesized that experimental mood induction (deliberately making subjects feel sad) would change interleukin (IL)-18 levels and N-opioid receptor availability. (IL-18 is a pro-inflammatory cytokine, a molecule that in several animal models increases the severity of disease[9]; N-opioid receptors bind receptor agonists like morphine producing sedation, analgesia, and in higher concentrations, euphoria.[10]

They utilized twenty-eight volunteers, half with MDD and half healthy individuals without MDD. They found that mood induction affected IL-18 (P @ 0.001) with sadness, increasing its levels, and neutral mood decreasing levels (P @ 0.001). Changes in IL-18 were more pronounced in the depressed volunteers (P = 0.03) and were linearly proportional to activation of M-opioid receptors by sadness. The conclusion was these data demonstrate dynamic changes in pro-inflammatory IL-1 superfamily cytokine IL-18 in response to experimentally induced sadness, which may delineate the role of neuroimmune interactions involving IL-18 in enhancing susceptibility to medical illnesses such as diabetes, heart disease, and persistent pain states in depressed individuals. (Where are the deep psychological conflicts in the deep unconscious in all of this?)

The gray matter of the brain contains the neurons, supportive cells,

---

[9] Interleukin-18, a pro-inflammatory cytokine, Dinarello, C. A. Eur. Cytokine Netw. 2000 Sep; 11 (3): 483–6.

[10] M-opioid receptor. From Wikipedia.

the dendrites and axons, and the synapses. It is distinguished from white matter consisting predominantly of myelinated axons. Gray matter is distributed in several areas of the brain, but consideration here will be given to the cerebral hemispheres. Gray matter, present in utero, undergoes substantial development and growth throughout childhood and adolescence. It is the major neural substrate responsible for muscle control, sensory perception, such as seeing and hearing, and the higher human capacities, memory, emotions, speech, decision-making, self-control, and mood regulation.

The normal trajectory of cortical gray matter in childhood proceeds with a burst of early neurogenesis and important increases in volume, resulting in thickening of the cortex. This has been associated with enhancement of cognitive and emotional functioning. At puberty, this first phase evolves into a second, in which a degree of pruning of neurons occurs for optimization of neuronal function and cognitive and emotional capacities.

Joan L. Luby et al.[11] were interested in determining if and how depression in early childhood impacted on cortical gray matter development. Their data was gathered in an academic research setting over an eleven-year period (September 2003 to December 2014); 193 children aged three to six years received behavioral assessments and MRI-imaging initially, which were repeated in the final phase of the study for comparison. Volume thickness and surface area of cortical gray matter were measured. Of the 193 children participating, 90 had a diagnosis of MDD. Findings demonstrated marked alterations of cortical gray matter, loss and thinning of it. They concluded the study demonstrated an association between early childhood depression and a trajectory of excessive pruning of neurons in childhood proportional to the severity of depressive symptoms, indicating they were losing

---

[11] "Early Childhood Depression and Alterations in the Trajectory of Gray Matter Maturation in Middle Childhood and Early Adolescence," Joan L. Luby, MD; Andy C. Belden, PhD; Joshua J. Jackson, PhD; Christina N. Lessov-Schlaggar, PhD; Michael P. Harms, PhD; Rebecca Tillman, MS; Kelly Botheron, MD; Diana Whalen, PhD; Deanna M. Barch, PhD, JAMA Psychiatry, Published online December 16, 2015.

gray matter at nearly twice the rate of unaffected peers—and that this accelerated loss of neurons started in childhood. Their results were consistent with prior studies of children diagnosed with schizophrenia and bipolar disorder showing an accelerated loss of gray matter, which can be interpreted as a form of premature brain aging.

Just think of it, preschool children with major depression losing neurons at an accelerated rate, undergoing a kind of nightmare of early lobotomy. And the lucky ones may receive mental health care treatment. Instead, it is urgent they be evaluated as early as possible by expert pediatric brain psychiatrists who are knowledgeable about the serious brain issues at stake and trained in administering sophisticated psychopharmacology to alleviate the attrition of vital brain tissue.

GLOSSARY

amygdale. A set of neurons linked to fear and pleasure responses.

anxiety disorders. Include generalized anxiety disorder, panic disorder, phobias, agoraphobia, and obsessive-compulsive disorder.

apoptosis. Programmed cell death.

atrophy. A wasting away of living tissue.

basal ganglia. A group of subcortical nuclei responsible primarily for motor control among other roles.

BDNF. A brain-derived neurotrophic factor.

cerebellum. A region at the posterior part of brain that is important for coordination of movement.

cingulate gyrus. Part of limbic system, which helps regulate emotion and pain.

cortex (cortical). The brain's outer layer, which contains neurons.

executive control. A set of brain processes that promote adaptation to the environment.

glucocorticoid receptors. Bind cortisol and other glucocorticoids.

glutamate. An amino acid neurotransmitter generally having excitatory effect on neurons.

glutamate toxicity. An excess of glutamate promotes damage to nerves, neurons, and glial cells.

glucocorticoid receptors. Bind cortisol and other glucocorticoids.

gray matter. The brain substance containing neurons.

hippocampus. The part of the brain involved in memory formation and memory storage. It is part of the limbic system.

limbic system. Set of brain structures buried under the cortex and involved in emotions and motivations.

meta-analysis. Using specialized statistical methods to get a pooled estimate of the results of individual scientific studies.

MRI imaging. A medical imaging technique used to visualize the anatomy and physiology of diseases.

neurotrophic factors. A family of biomolecules that are peptides or small proteins that support neuron health.

orbital frontal cortex. Prefrontal cortex region involved in cognitive processing and decision-making.

pathological alterations. Histopathological abnormalities in body tissue, sometimes requiring examination with a microscope to identify.

receptors. Structures in cell membranes where communication molecules dock to set off a signal in the receiving cell.

steroid hormones. They help control metabolism, inflammation, immune functions, salt and water balance, and sexual characteristics.

synapses. The delicate structures through which neurons communicate with one another utilizing neurotransmitters.

thalamus. A body of neurons that relay sensory information from receptors to the brain.

volumetric reductions. Loss of brain tissue, atrophy.

working memory. A core executive function necessary to stay focused and coordinate information.

CHAPTER 4

Robin Williams

On August 12, 2014, "Robin Williams is Dead at Age 63" appeared in the *Wall Street Journal*. In the article, the apparent cause of death as suicide by asphyxiation is noted, and the fact he had publicly discussed his struggles with alcohol and drug addiction. Depression is not mentioned. Was he ever given a thorough evaluation by an experienced medically oriented psychiatrist practiced in clinical psychopharmacology? Was he being prescribed an appropriate regime of medications, often in combination, and closely monitored? It appears he was sober at the time of the final suicidal act. What really killed him remains in the shadows. It's as if he instead had a cough and then died, and his death was attributed to the cough and not an underlying untreated pneumonia. As an afterthought, it was subsequently mentioned he had been diagnosed with Parkinson's disease. If he had been, it was most likely in a very early phase of that disease, which would not be fatal.

Robin McLaurin Williams was born on July 21, 1951, in Chicago. Before college, he initially decided to study political science but then, having a dramatic change of heart, enrolled at the Julliard School to study theater. There, along with Christopher Reeve, he was selected for the school's advanced program in dramatic training. After he left Julliard, he first performed in nightclubs where he was discovered for the role of Mork on an episode of *Happy Days* in 1974, which subsequently became *Mork and Mindy* in 1978. Over the next 36 years, countless millions were amused, entertained, made hilarious or brought to tears by his dramatic and comic genius. He won an Oscar, two Emmys, two SAG Awards, six Golden Globes and six Grammys. For this author, the images and antics of *Mrs. Doubtfire* still bring feelings of amusement, pleasure, and warmth. Mr. Williams was a lovable treasure of a man.

His wife, Susan Schneider, wanted her statement run in its entirety at the time of his death. His daughter, Robin, took solace after his death from the tremendous outpouring of affection and admiration for him. He had touched millions of lives. Sorrowfully, she commented, "I'll never understand how he could be loved so deeply and not find it in his heart to stay."

Robin Williams went out of his way to intervene in the lives of ordinary individuals who were struggling with difficult personal circumstances. A teenage cancer patient made an educational piece for television with him. Her mother noted, "They danced for hours as he joked and made her laugh all day. Robin Williams is very kind-hearted and an incredible soul." He was recently diagnosed with early Parkinson's disease. A close friend, Michael J. Fox, had been stunned to hear about the diagnosis. However, early Parkinson's disease usually does not present an imminent danger to one so diagnosed. Mr. Fox had received his diagnosis in 1991, and he was still continuing to act in several roles at the time of Williams's death.

On August 11, 2014, an article with photos appeared on Radar Online. Williams had been attending rehab at Hazelden Addiction Treatment Center in Minnesota. He was described as gaunt. According to a Dairy Queen employee with whom he was photographed, he was subdued and unrecognizable. "I didn't think it was actually him at first," she commented. Judging from his visage in the photograph and an apparent depletion of his verbalizations and probable diminishment of his body activity and movements, it is probable he was demonstrating symptoms of severe major depression with psychomotor retardation. It is not known if a detailed assessment was made to rule out major depression or if he was prescribed antidepressant medications. At any rate, a month later, he was dead.

Shortly after his personal assistant arrived at his home, she became concerned because he had failed to respond to knocks on the door. She discovered him in his room, a belt around his neck, suspended from a door. Although his addiction problems are highlighted and he was battling his demons, the role of depression is underplayed. This is not at all surprising. It is all too easy to trivialize and diminish the role of a so-called mental illness. Indeed, the early Parkinson's diagnosis is given more attention. (After all, it's a physical illness.) The high likelihood is that clinical depression, not early Parkinson's disease, resulted in his death by suicide.

The key question then is, can depression kill and do so on an involuntary basis? And if so, by what mechanisms? Are there physical brain abnormalities in clinical depression as there are in neurological illnesses of the brain (seizure disorders, multiple sclerosis, amyolateral sclerosis)? Are there abnormalities of thinking and emotion that undergo a phase change in which suicidal thoughts and emotions become the immobile components of abnormal physical-like processes and structures in the brain that freeze the suicidal ideations as if in ice or concrete, leaving these thoughts and emotions beyond the control of willpower? And what is the content of these frozen thoughts and the nature of the emotions they are linked to?

First, the brain itself. Clinical depression has now been studied by the latest technology available. What was invisible has become visible, available to the scrutiny of cutting-edge science employing MRI (magnetic resonance imaging). A selective review[12] of all T1-weighted structural MRI studies published between 2000 and 2007 found patients with major depressive disorder had (physical) structural brain abnormalities. There were volumetric reductions in several major brain areas including the hippocampus, basal ganglia, and orbital and frontal cortex. In other words, when compared to the same studies of individuals not having major depressive disorder,

---

[12] *A Journal of Affective Disorders* 117 (2009), 1–17.

the respective brain areas were smaller than normal. (This would be consistent with damage to these areas with resultant atrophy of them due to the abnormal regression and death of brain cells [neurons] during development.)

The process of a neuron dying is called apoptosis. Obviously, something more than mental is going on if the disease of major depression provokes the death of neurons relative to individuals who do not have major depression. These extensive scientific studies demonstrate pathologic alterations of extensive brain areas, both cortical and limbic; the extent of the injury is generally proportional to the severity of the major depressive illness.

A reduction in gray matter density refers to a decrease in the number of neurons and supporting cells in a given volume of gray matter, which is the fundamental type of brain tissue in important brain areas, the orbital frontal cortex, cingulate gyrus, cerebellum, and thalamus. It is responsible for general intellectual ability, executive control of attention, working memory, and decision-making, which are all critical for functioning successfully in society. As already noted, major depressive disorder does lead to apoptosis in those areas, which can impact the quality and efficiency of these functions. The level of reduced function is proportional to the intensity of apoptosis.

Apoptosis is the process in which neurons literally commit suicide. Some neuron apoptosis is part of normal development in the fetus between conception and birth, a kind of pruning on behalf of brain efficiency. In adult years, apoptosis is triggered by genes, which if activated, promote neurons to self-destruct. Dozens of neurotropic factors regulate the continued survival of neurons. Other neurotropic factors when genetically triggered cause neurons to suicide. It is scientifically beyond dispute that the severe so-called mental illnesses promote apoptosis. Two prominent mechanisms involve the suppression of BDNF (brain-derived neurotropic factor), which plays a critical role in the proper growth and maintenance of neurons, and the excess production of glutamate, which excites neurons to death, but at normal levels, it is an important neurotransmitter. Both these paths to neuron death are operative in so-called mental illnesses.

The Hippocampus

This important area, which in isolation resembles a seahorse, historically was considered to be involved in olfaction (smell). However, more recently, it has been considered to have three main functions. First, it is important in maintaining impulse control, the inhibition of responses that could be excessive, inappropriate, or self-destructive. In other words, it is a metaphorical brake on dysfunctional behavior. It assists in maintaining more quiet, adaptive behavioral responses. A second major function relates to memory, particularly forming new memories as well as playing a role in explicitly verbalizing memories acquired through experiences, memories, and facts. A third function may have bearing on aspects of the symptom of anxiety. It takes little imagination to see how structural abnormalities and neuron loss (apoptosis) can lead to significant symptoms.

There is a reliable relationship between the size of the hippocampus and memory performance. For example, elderly people who show hippocampal shrinkage (not all elderly people do) perform significantly less well on tests of memory. Another route that can impair memory does not require the actual loss of neurons, but of the connections between them (synapses). This subtler physical damage also occurs during severe, so-called mental illnesses. A major factor in hippocampal damage is related to high levels of glucocorticoid receptors in the hippocampus. The major so-called mental illnesses are generally associated with high levels of emotional stress and the release of excess levels of steroid hormones. This is true for severe major depression, post-traumatic stress disorder, bipolar disorders, schizophrenia, and severe anxiety disorders. Because the hippocampus is heavily populated with receptors for the stress hormones, destructive biological processes occur, leading to hippocampal shrinkage and atrophy in all these illnesses.

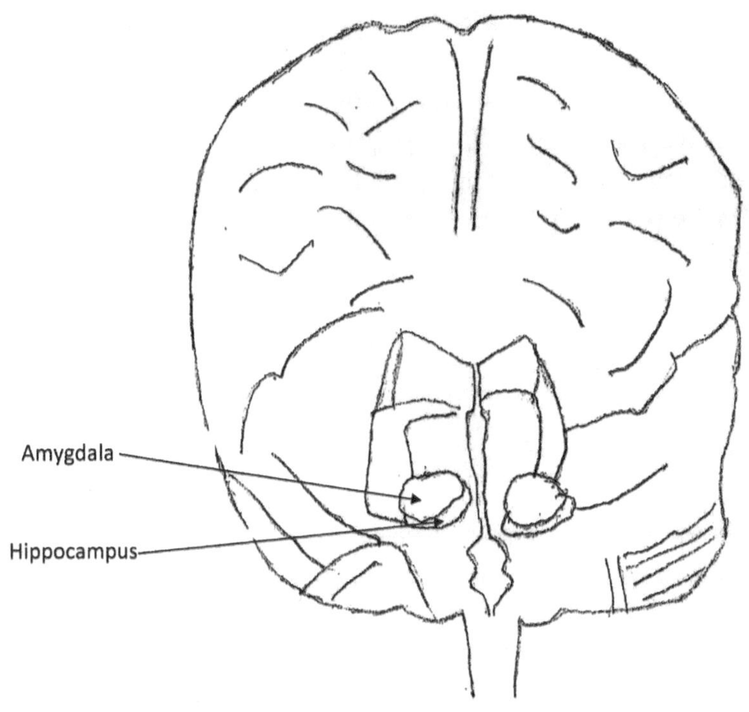

The Human Brain - The Amygdala and Hippocampus

It should be only too clear how physical all this is, but psychiatry still calls the above-mentioned illnesses mental. In psychology, denying reality to the point of total illogicality and blindness to facts is called psychosis. Perhaps calling so-called mental illnesses mental illnesses represents a psychosis in itself. Actually, perhaps individuals who label other people mentally ill, particularly psychiatrists, are the actual ones with mental illness! When you think of it, that is the truth! They are also sadistic! Back to the hippocampus. Another group of illnesses classified as physical—convulsive disorders—also damage this same important brain part.

"The Hippocampus in Depression: A Meta-Analysis of MRI

Studies" by Paul Vidobech, MD, Barbara Ravnkilde, PhD, was published in the *American Journal of Psychiatry* in 2004. A meta-analysis is a scientific statistical technique to study and summarize the results of individual scientific studies in order to obtain the best possible scientific conclusions from the individual studies. The purpose of the studies in this case was to elucidate the relationship of major depressive illness to the size of the hippocampus. The question of whether depression is associated with shrinkage of the hippocampus is important to understanding the disease, and the relationship to the number of episodes and the magnitude of the shrinkage is similarly important. Twelve scientific studies were of sufficient quality to be included in the meta-analysis. The MRIs of 351 patients with major depression were carefully compared with the MRIs of 279 healthy controls (people who did not have a history or symptoms of major depression). The effect of the illness and the size of the hippocampus was conclusive. There was a 10 percent reduction of the right hippocampus in the patients, and if there was a history of reoccurring episodes of illness, the shrinkage increased. There was a smaller degree of shrinkage of the left hippocampus. There is a hopeful aspect, some evidence that antidepressant medications can stop hippocampal atrophy and/or reduce it. It is hypothesized that antidepressants promote neurogenesis (the birth of new neurons) in addition to previous discussed positive influences on neurotropic factors and reduction of glutamate toxicity. In order to reduce hippocampal shrinkage, the importance of early institution of treatment with antidepressant medication and supportive therapy becomes very clear!

The Amygdalae

For such a relatively small brain region in size, the amygdalae are involved with many important brain functions, and damage to them is connected to a variety of debilitating symptoms. As is the case with the hippocampus, multiple MRI studies have been conducted to compare the amygdalae size and structure of patients with MDD to those of normal controls without the illness. Patients with the illness have significant reduction in size.

Some studies have shown children with anxiety disorders tend to have a smaller left amygdala. The left amygdala has been linked with social anxiety disorder, obsessive-compulsive disorder, and post-traumatic stress disorder. Patients with more severe social anxiety disorder show a correlation with excessive activity in the amygdala. Similarly, patients with major depression demonstrate increased activity there also. It is a picture of the important brain part being somewhat shrunken but also hyperactive and overexcitable. Again, this is a physical and not a mental phenomenon. Structural and functional abnormalities of the amygdalae are not under voluntary control and have widespread emotional and cognitive consequences.

As mentioned, the amygdalae are multifunctional by means of their own divisions and their interconnectedness with other brain regions. They play an important role in decision-making and taking action. Larger amygdalae are correlated with the capacity for making better social judgments, enabling greater societal integration and cooperation. Conversely, smaller amygdalae are associated with social and emotional deficits. They play a role in processing both negative and positive emotions.

On the negative side, fear, sadness, anger, and the poor regulation of aggression are symptoms. On the contrary side, they can generate feelings of happiness and accomplishments. They play a major role in the processing of memory, especially ones with a significant emotional component. They select which memories to keep and what part of the brain to assign them to for storage and consolidate them for later recall of relevant details. Larger amygdalae tend to be associated with greater creativity. Monkey mothers with smaller amygdalae tend to neglect and treat their infants harshly. The amygdalae are not above performing more basic bodily functions, playing a role in heart rate and blood pressure equilibration.

Gray Matter Entities, the Orbital Frontal Cortex, and the Prefrontal Cortex

The more severe so-called mental illnesses negatively impact the gray matter of the brain. The cerebral cortex, the gray matter of the surface of the brain, is arranged in a sort of hill-and-crevice pattern. In this gray matter resides the neurons, supporting cells, and the vessels for the supply of blood. Our essential humanity, that entity which is ourselves, our awareness, our identity, and our reasoning abilities dwell within the gray matter. In the most severe so-called mental illnesses, in which there has been little or no effective treatment received, there can be widespread thinning and depletion of its substance, corresponding to widespread apoptosis (neuron suicide).

The Cerebral Cortex is grey matter and constitutes the lobes of the brain

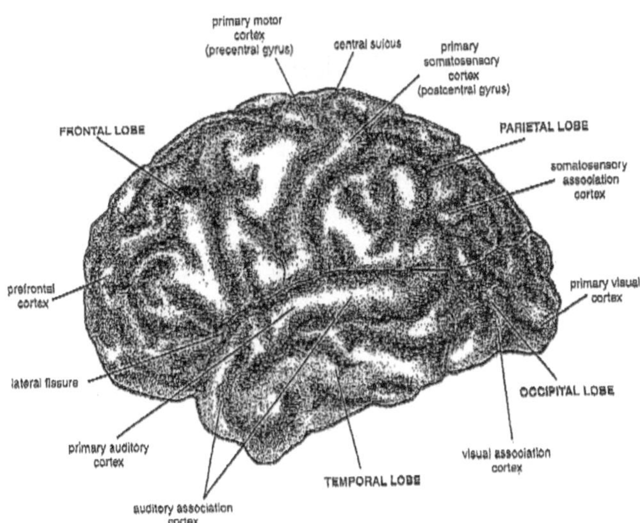

Key brain regions. This is a simple visual representation f the localization of several key regions of the cerebral cortex. The frontal lobe comprises the cortical area in front of the central suicus, while the prefrontal cortex is the subregion of the frontal lobe in front of the primary motor cortex. The other lobes – parietal, temporal, and occipital – are also shown. Auditory areas are primarily located in the temporal lobes; visual areas are in the occipital lobe, and somatosensory areas in the parietal lobe.

The Orbital Frontal Cortex

A part of the cerebral cortex—the prefrontal cortex division of it—resides immediately above the orbits of the eyes. It plays a primary role in the selection of actions to implement. It estimates expected rewards/punishments of an action selected and processes the execution of the action, whereupon it calibrates an actual result of the action against the previous estimation of the result. It plays an important role in motivational drives and modifications, reinforcing certain actions and behaviors. It is critical for adoptive learning. It has connectivity with the hippocampus, the amygdalae, and additional brain regions. When the orbital-frontal cortex and connections are disrupted, varying degrees of cognitive, emotional, and behavioral impairments ensue.

Was Robin Williams's life lost for no particular reason? Did he hang himself as part of a comedy routine? Did he have a wisp of some mental problem that didn't even warrant an evaluation and treatment by a professional who was knowledgeable enough to make a competent diagnosis and experienced enough to provide scientific evidence-based treatment? It certainly doesn't seem so! He was a victim of the treacherous dichotomy, in which so-called mental illnesses are trivialized by most people, most therapists, most physicians, and most therapy psychiatrists. Isn't it likely he had actual abnormalities of his brain—physical brain abnormalities consistent with major depression? Did anybody, particularly so-called mental health professionals—if he was evaluated by one—ever consider that, let alone provide targeted, appropriate treatment? (It will be necessary to discuss what such treatment should be for the brain illness underlying the symptoms of major depression).

In 2016, Susan Schneider Williams wrote a letter about her husband's suicide in *Neurology*). It was called "The Terrorist inside My Husband's Brain." In it, she states her belief his suicide was precipitated as a response to a severe neurological disease, Lewy body disease (LBD), which was only diagnosed in the autopsy. Intra-neuronal abnormal proteins called Lewy bodies were identified in his neurons.

In the article, she relates the grueling procession of symptoms she had observed. There were at first more general symptoms, constipation, urinary difficulty, heartburn, and then sleeplessness. His sense of smell was poor, and he developed a slight tremor in his left hand. His fear and anxiety skyrocketed, which was out of character for him. She began to wonder if he was a hypochondriac, but she was reassured when she learned LBD could cause severe anxiety symptoms. After several months, he developed problems with paranoia, delusions, memory dysfunction, and high cortisol levels, but she was relieved when she learned Lewy bodies within the amygdala could cause these out-of-character symptoms. The symptoms were not an indication of weakness in his heart, spirit, or character. Next, he developed panic attacks. She was enormously upset when it became apparent even though, his fears were unfounded, she no longer could convince him otherwise.

> He had reached a place we had never been before. My husband was trapped in the twisted architecture of his neurons. Brain scans were normal, the only lab abnormality, the elevated cortisol. Then Parkinson's disease (PD) was diagnosed. At last, a label had been put on his enormous distress and suffering. The Parkinson's disease was characterized as mild, although over time, symptoms progressed. His left-hand tremor became continuous; he developed a slow, shuffling gait, had word-finding difficulties, changes in his visual and spatial abilities, and loss of basic reasoning.

She noted a history of depression six years previously, but when he showed signs of depression starting about six months before his death, it was interpreted as a satellite issue, maybe connected to his PD. He continued to be delusional and developed hallucinations. He was treated with medication for PD, but there is no mention of pharmacological treatment for major depression—let alone sophisticated, competent treatment for severe psychotic major depressive episode.

His widow closes by expressing her appreciation for neurology. "However you look at it—the presence of Lewy bodies took his life." She expresses her hope neurological science will find an answer so others will not have to suffer like Robin.

What is striking is the total minimization of a possible role in his symptomatic suffering and suicide of a severe mood disorder in association with the neurological illness, as if this would not be an acceptable etiology for his suicide or a contributing factor to it. She wishes she had the chance to tell him his suffering and suicide were caused by Lewy body disease.

Lewy body disease is a real physical brain illness, and not a mental problem.

Mrs. Williams cannot be blamed for dichotomizing. The blame sits firmly in the lap of organized psychiatry, which perpetuates the dichotomy. They specialize in treating mental problems and are immune from the neuroscientific evidence that the major so-called mental problems are physical brain disorders. This adds fuel to the burden of stigmatization, trivialization, and denial.

CHAPTER 5

Phineas Gage

According to *Smithsonian,* Jack and Beverly Wilgus, collectors of nineteenth-century versions of daguerreotypes came across one of a disfigured yet still handsome man. There were no clues about who he was, when it was taken, or why he was holding a substantial tapered metal rod. They assumed he must have been sailor engaged in whale hunting. In December 2007, they posted the photograph on the internet and received a reply that the rod was not a harpoon—and that he probably had not been in the whaling trade.

Another informant suggested the individual was Phineas Gage,[13] who had a very unique history in the study of the brain. He had been a foreman of a crew of railroad construction workers. In 1848, at the age of twenty-five, he was preparing to set up an explosion by drilling a hole in rock. He was tamping in the explosive powder with an iron rod when a spark set off the explosion prematurely, sending the rod at high speed straight through his skull. It entered his left cheek, exited the top of his head, and landed thirty yards away. He was transported by wagon to his boardinghouse and examined by Dr. Harlow. His wounds were dressed but not treated surgically.

During the initial treatment and the follow-up evaluations, Dr. Harlow made a number of observations. Gage retained full possession

---

[13] "Phineas Gage: Neuroscience's Most Famous Patient," Steve Twomey, Smithsonian.com, Jan. 2010.

of his reason after the accident, but others closest to him—his wife, relatives, and friends—began to notice changes in his personality. It wasn't until twenty years later, in 1868, that Dr. Harlow made a formal report in the *Bulletin of The Massachusetts Medical Society*:

> His contractors, who regarded him as the most efficient and capable foreman in their employ previous to his injury, considered the change in his mind so marked that they could not give him his place again. He was described fitful, irreverent, indulging at times in the grossest profanity (which was not previously his custom), manifesting but little deference for his fellows, impatient of restraint of advice when it conflicts with his desires, at times pertinaciously obstinate, yet capricious and vacillating, devising many plans of future operation, which are no sooner arranged than they are abandoned in turn for others appearing more feasible. In this regard, his mind was radically changed, so decidedly that his friends and acquaintances said he was no longer Gage.

It became apparent that damage to the frontal cortex was associated with loss of social inhibitions and with inappropriate behavior. There is controversy about the quality of his life from the time of the accident until his death in San Francisco in 1860. His brother-in-law exhumed his skull and sent it to Dr. Harlow who donated it to Harvard Medical School where it now resides at Warren Anatomy Museum in Boston (along with the iron rod). Cavendish, a small town in Vermont closest to where the accident occurred, built a memorial plaque for him in 1999.

As already noted, the earliest conceptions of the role of the prefrontal cortex were in serving as an integral linkage to a person's personality and the expression of it. With the advent of modern neuroscience, its immense complexity in forming the essence of human capabilities and intelligence has become apparent. It consists of the cortical granular layer (containing neurons, associated cells, and blood vessels), which account for the first third of the outermost layer of the brain. It maintains connections with nearly every other part of the brain.

In thinking about the prefrontal cortex, it can be useful to use a metaphor: the brain's master panel. It incorporates and represents information from the environment and information from multiple brain areas, formulating all the inputs into a coherent whole, essentially to permit survival and adaptation in a whole spectrum of external and internal environments. Thoughts and potential actions and emotions are represented, inputted from multiple brain areas, and evaluated for their appropriateness and anticipated results in relation to formulated objectives and goals.

A degree of inhibition is maintained until potentially inappropriate responses can be suppressed and appropriate responses are made ready to be allowed into the environment. Once expressed, the results of the action are measured against what was previously anticipated. A subset of the master panel deals with the social realm, a similar testing of what will be appropriate social responses versus inappropriate ones, and corresponding assessment of the feedback.

It is the repository of planning, decision-making, and determination of appropriate social behavior. The prefrontal cortex also maintains arousal, awareness, and sentience. It has the prominent role in mediating normal sleep physiology and dreaming. A particularly interesting function of a particular part, the medial prefrontal cortex, spends its time thinking about and analyzing the attributes of other individuals. Most importantly, a well-functioning prefrontal cortex is a necessity for accurately determining reality. Several studies have indicated that reduced volume and interconnections of the frontal lobes with other brain regions is observed in severe so-called mental illness. The symptoms that are derived from it, unfortunately, are found in many of the more disabling illnesses: severe sleep disturbances, difficulties in functioning and decision-making, interrupted concentration, inability to persist toward goals important for their well-being, poor self-esteem, difficulties in relationships, loneliness, and social isolation.

Gage likely had many or most of these symptoms. He must have been mentally ill. The iron rod passing through his brain must have been a *mental* metal rod!

CHAPTER 6

A Neural Model of Major Depressive Disorder

The neurological illnesses—stroke, multiple sclerosis, epilepsy, Parkinson's disease, and others—have long been classified as physical or *real* illnesses because definite physical abnormalities (even biochemical ones) could be associated with the symptoms. Into a dark hole went the so-called mental illnesses because no similar brain abnormalities were in evidence. In spite of evidence these illnesses could be associated with massive suffering, disability, and death, they were cast adrift into their own separate category, exclaiming they are indeed mental illnesses.

A real physical illness elicits understandable sympathy, understanding, and support, but the sufferer of a so-called mental illness must live with the constant suspicion that others may doubt they are really ill or really suffering. Some resolution, determination, willpower, and a trifle less self-pity and laziness would swing the equilibrium back to health—if they would only get off it and get going!

At last an exhaustive scientific study utilized MRI analysis after centuries of suffering compounded by humiliation and punishment. What had been invisible has become visible, revealing structural physical abnormalities in the brains of people with so-called mental illness.

First, a brief comment on the scientific method. In order for a study, experiment, or investigation to be termed *scientific*, inquiry must be based on objectively measured evidence gathered systematically, with principles employed to avoid bias and personal opinion from contaminating the conclusions, which are eventually drawn forth from the data gathered in the study. All the data, methodologies, and conclusions must be available for careful scrutiny by other scientists and qualified professionals.

In a very large study, "Functional Neuroimaging of Major Depressive Disorders," investigators reviewed the entire scientific literature up to 2012 for individual studies employing neuroimaging (MRI, PET, and SPECT scans) of patients with major depressive disorder and matched individuals who did not have the illness (labeled normal controls or healthy.) All in all, they found 6,595 such studies.

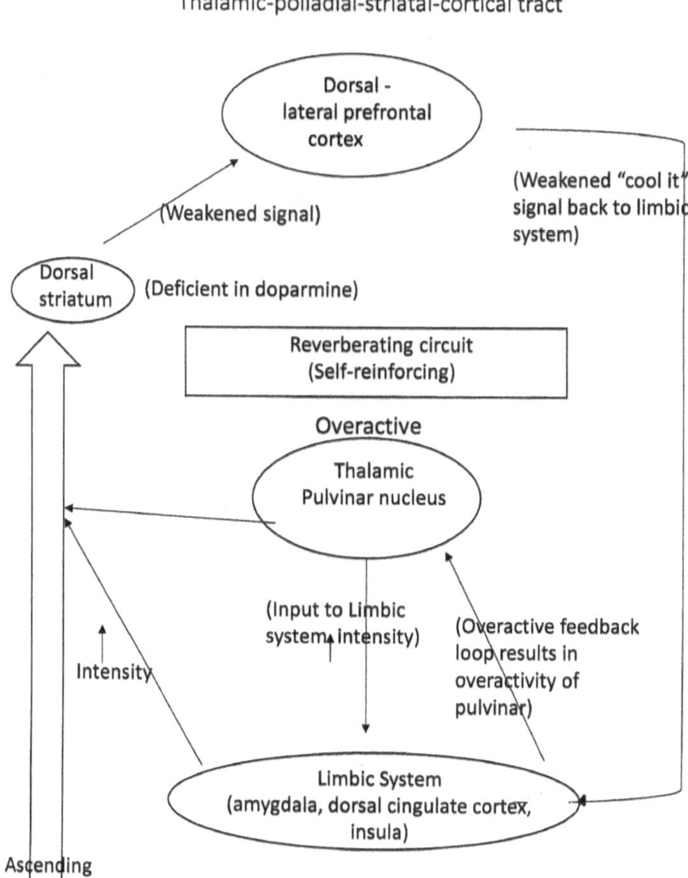

Through a laborious winnowing process, they finally selected the best forty studies. These forty studies were entered into the meta-analysis, which is a quantitative statistical analysis applied to all the studies, pooling the data to test the effectiveness of the results. All the included studies in the meta-analysis were of the whole brain, aiming to visualize the brain in detail to examine baseline levels of activation in relevant brain structures and neural reactivity to both positive and negative stimuli. The meta-analysis can yield findings not apparent in any single study, identifying abnormal patterns of activation and abnormal responses to both positive and negative stimuli. The ultimate objective of this laborious process was to develop a neuroanatomically viable model of MDD in the living brain of those suffering from the disease and compare those findings with the findings of the matching data of those who did not have the disease.

There follows a schematic presentation of the findings allowing tolerance for the fact the author is a clinician and not a neuroscientist who is trying his best to relay the results.

First a brief note on brain structure, brain cells (neurons), and their connectivity. Neurons are physical structures often gathered in dense pockets called nuclei. The connecting wires between neurons are the axons and dendrites.

From the meta-analytic synthesis, it was possible to formulate as accurate a model as possible using the latest scientific data from whole brain neuroimaging studies of patients with MDD and matching controls without the disease.

The Findings:

Insert illustration, Fig. 3 Neural Model of Biased Responding to Negative Information in Major Depressive Disorder.

A large nucleus in the thalamus, the pulvinar nucleus has a higher level of baseline activity than in normal controls. The pulvinar nucleus sends its signals by its projections (axons) to additional regions in the limbic system: the amygdala, dorsal anterior cingulate cortex, and the insula, which return negative feedback to the pulvinar nucleus. This creates a self-reinforcing excess state of stimulation in this limbic system nexus. This is likely an important mechanism for symptoms of severe clinical anxiety and emotional and mood volatility many people with so-called mental illness are liable to.

This reverberating circuit also has important connections to an ascending pathway moving up to the dorsal striatum and finally the dorsolateral prefrontal cortex. The name of the ascending track is the *thalamic-palladial-striatal-cortical.* Unfortunately for those with MDD, there is a deficiency of the neurotransmitter dopamine in the striatum and its nigral subcomponent. Because of this, the signal that is supposed to be sent to the dorsolateral prefrontal cortex is seriously attenuated and its function significantly impaired. The dorsolateral prefrontal cortex performs the rational functions of evaluating the fear from the limbic system, applying appropriate perspectives and rational reappraisals, and after doing so, sending signals back to the hyperactive limbic network to cool it. Because the limbic input from the ascending track is weakened by dopamine deficiency, resulting in a weakened signal to the dorsolateral prefrontal cortex, this attenuates the positive feedback loop from it back to the overstimulated limbic system, and the latter is left in an unmodulated dysfunctional state.

Theorists have long contended that biased processing of negative information plays a central role in the etiology and maintenance of major depressive illness. The researchers by dint of great effort, patience, and scientific expertise have been able to formulate the underlying neural dysfunctions, especially the enhanced processing of negative information that is the fundamental etiology and cause of major depressive illness.

The researchers have also noted antidepressant medications, if properly titrated to effective dosage levels, give evidence of correcting the aforementioned anomalous mechanisms.

A Neuron

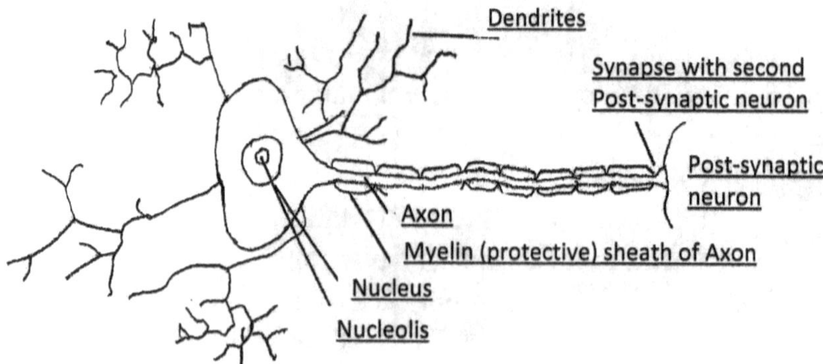
Dendrites
Synapse with second
Post-synaptic neuron
Post-synaptic
neuron
Axon
Myelin (protective) sheath of Axon
Nucleus
Nucleolis

GLOSSARY

cell membrane. A biological membrane separating the interior of cells from the outside environment.

coding region of gene. Regulating region of gene that determines if a particular gene will be activated.

lysosome. A membrane-bound organelle in the cell's cytoplasm that releases enzymes for cellular processes.

neurogenesis. Process by which neurons are generated from neural stem cells.

organelles. Specialized subunits in a cell. Examples are the Golgi apparatus, lysosomes, and endoplasmic reticulum.

ribosomes. The protein manufacturers of the cell. They are complex molecular machines.

RNA. Ribonucleic acid is a macromolecule directing flow of genetic information from DNA to outside the nucleus to manufacture proteins.

SNP. A single-nucleotide polymorphism. Each SNP represents a single DNA building block, a nucleotide.

synaptogenesis. The formation of synapses between neurons.

vesicle. Small fluid-filled sac delivering critical molecules where required in the cell.

CHAPTER 7

The Neuron

It is the neurons, the specialized cells of the human brain, and in particular their interconnectedness, that form the infrastructure that accounts for all manifestations of human intelligence, but also the dysfunctions, which lead to the disorders and diseases of the brain, neurological illnesses, and major so-called mental illnesses.

The treacherous dichotomy is nonexistent in the actual, real physical brain. There is not a physical cause for physical brain illnesses (seizure disorders, multiple sclerosis, myasthenia gravis, or stroke) and mental causes for so-called mental illnesses (severe major depression, panic disorder, obsessive compulsive disorder, or schizophrenia). The psychiatric profession, which professes to be expert on unconscious motivation and processes, is a primary perpetuator of the treacherous dichotomy. The majority of psychiatrists categorize themselves as therapists and are deeply invested in the maintenance of the treacherous dichotomy. Many therapy psychiatrists may help some people but they consciously (and unconsciously) classify them as mentally ill. And first do no harm (*primum non nocere*)! Psychiatrists, like most human beings, protect that which butters their bread, in their case administering weekly forty-five-minute psychotherapy.

About 20 percent of psychiatrists adhere to a more medical orientation. They emphasize studying the brain and its physical construction. (For example, studying and digesting a text like *Stahl's*

Essential Psychopharmacology, Neuroscientific Basis and Practical Applications.) In other words, they behave like real physicians, that is like neurologists, the other medical specialty that treats brain illnesses. Neurologists adhere strongly to the medical model. They do not neglect their medical responsibilities to perform physical therapy; they refer to nonmedical specialists to do that.

As we learn more and more about the brain, it is abundantly clear psychiatry as a profession cannot perpetually straddle the fence. The fork in the road is here now! Either choose a therapist or a medical specialist who is knowledgeable about the physical malfunctions of the brain. The patient's dilemma is to know which is which, the therapy psychiatrist from the brain psychiatrist. The latter learns about the brain and the specific physical mechanisms, which when malfunctioning, cause the symptoms of so-called mental illness. Through skillful use of corrective medications, they are most likely to promote reductions in symptoms, suffering, and disability.

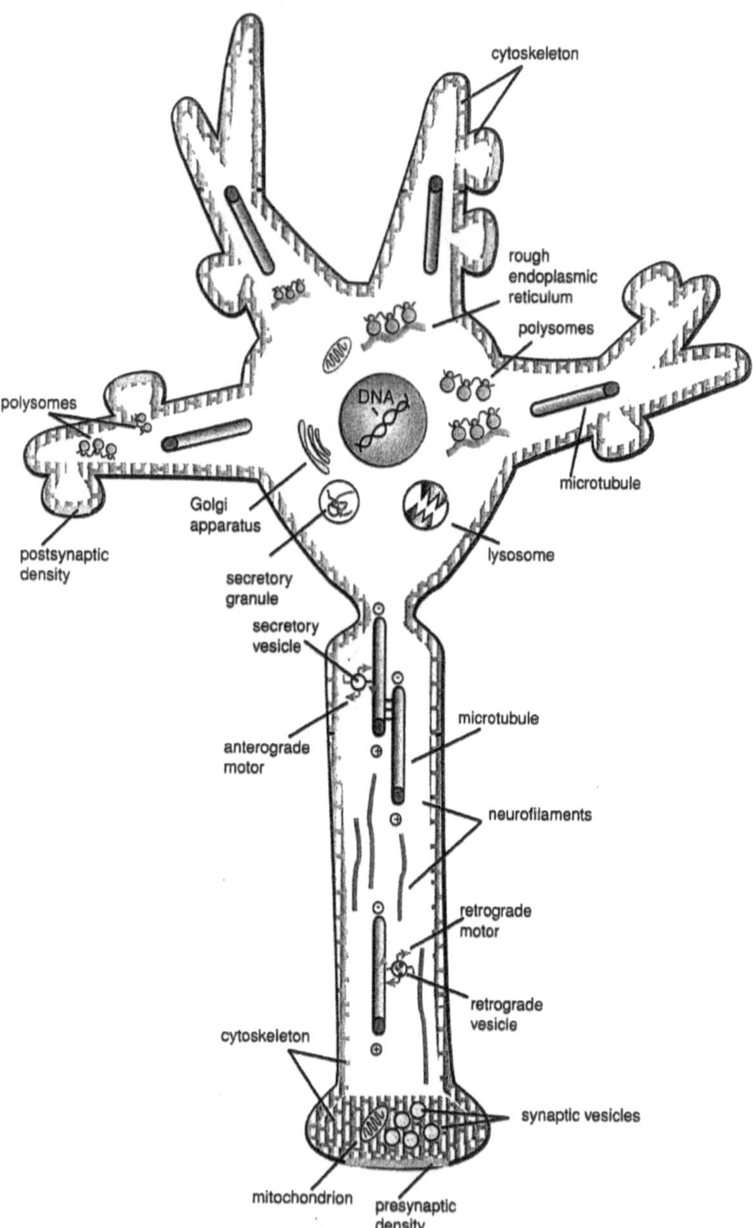
Localization of Subcellular Organelles
cytoskeleton
rough
endoplasmic
reticulum
polysomes
polysomes
DNA
microtubule
Golgi
apparatus
lysosome
postsynaptic
density
secretory
granule
secretory
vesicle
microtubule
anterograde
motor
neurofilaments
retrograde
motor
retrograde
vesicle
cytoskeleton
synaptic vesicles
mitochondrion
presynaptic
density

Localization of Subcellular Organelles

The neuron is an invisible and microscopic intricate, elaborate, detailed living machine. Its multiple synergistically functioning components, when multiplied into the 100 billion neurons of the entire brain, constitute the infrastructure for human intelligence and creativity, but also when in a state of dysfunction, result in brain diseases. In identical fashion, the so-called mental illnesses, understanding neuronal functions and structure as well as dysfunction is an important basis for comprehending these brain disorders.

A neuron's main task is to create a signal that is meant to communicate with other neurons. Essentially, the neuron comes into existence by a process of manufacturing itself. Its genes contain elaborate instructions for the self-manufacture to proceed. It must manufacture all its working parts (organelles) and build the scaffolding that provides a secure structure that contains them.

To manufacture its body, the genes send out RNA molecules from the nucleus to the manufacturing centers, the polysomes, and endoplasmic reticulum, which according to the instructions, manufacture specialized proteins, which consist of the cytoskeleton, microtubules, neurofilaments, and presynaptic densities. The first stage of manufacture occurs through the action at the endoplasmic reticulum. The partially manufactured components are packaged into vesicles and transported to the Golgi apparatus, which applies the finishing touches, completing the manufacturing process of the cytoskeleton components, microtubules, neurofilaments, and density proteins, which are again packaged into vesicles to be transported to their final destinations in the neuron.

The express anterograde transport system conveys mitochondria, synaptic vesicles, growth factors, anterograde secretory vesicles, retrograde secretory vesicles, receptors, enzymes, ion channels, neurotransmitters, reuptake pumps, and peptides. The slow transport system carries the slow and fast transport motors themselves, cytoplasmic protein microtubules, cytoskeleton elements, and neurofilaments.

In order to reach their final destinations, these structural components must be transported to them. For this, the transport systems spring into action. The anterograde is the one with motors, which latch onto the vesicles and actively move them (like little trucks). There are, of course, a sufficient number of motors to get the job done. In the illustration, one anterograde motor is moving a microtubule out of the cell body, down the axon, dropping it off as it goes to provide inner structure and support for the axon at the proper location. There are actually two delivery systems that transport needed parts. The express travels really fast at 200 mm per day (a huge distance considering the neuron is dramatically smaller than 1 mm), and the slow at a fraction of that speed.

From this long list of vital components the neuron requires to function properly, it is clear what an intricate little living machine it is!

Of course, components wear out, so they must be transported back into the cell body and brought to the lysosomes for destruction. Another transport system provides for this. The retrograde, which is only half as fast as the anterograde system, travels 100 mm per day. All the components just listed require first being manufactured, and when useful life is over, transport back for destruction.

Neurotransmitters are the one component of the neuron that people may be familiar with. Serotonin has made it into the lay press, and many are aware it is a well-being neurotransmitter. It also must be manufactured according to instructions from the genes in the nucleus, transported by fast-transport motors along the entire length of the axon to be stored in synaptic vesicles. When the neuron's signal passes down the axon, the vesicles containing it discharge the serotonin molecule through the end of the axon into the space just beyond it, the synaptic space, so they can dock on the receptors (little docks) of the next neuron (the postsynaptic neuron). The presynaptic neuron tries to conserve serotonin as much as possible, so the reuptake pumps actively transport unused serotonin back into the axon, prepackaging it for subsequent discharge.

In summary, understanding the structure and function of neurons is central to understanding (and competently treating) all physical brain disorders, including the neurological illnesses and the so-called mental illnesses. The essential unit of causation of both is the physical dysfunction of physical neurons. Therapy psychiatrists are not yet claiming there are mental neurons inhabiting the id, superego, and ego, but their researchers are hell-bent on proving that. Unfortunately (or fortunately), they are having great difficulty obtaining funds for that research.

Apoptosis

Apoptosis is the name given to a built-in program by which the neuron, on a signal from its genes, turns on a process that triggers its own destruction. In the forming brain, a careful form of apoptosis trims away redundant neurons. In the adult brain, small degrees of apoptosis in response to multiple stresses may be triggered. More specifically, in the case of physical neurons, environmental factors, diseases, trauma, insufficient oxygen, strokes, poisons, aging, and neurological disorders can trigger the apoptosis genes. Therapy psychiatry researchers are hard at work to elucidate the etiology of apoptosis in the case of mental neurons in illnesses such as severe major depression, bipolar disorder, obsessive-compulsive disorder, and schizophrenia. A leading hypothesis is that crazy or dirty thoughts cause apoptosis in these mental illnesses.

Neuronal Migration

The brain has a complex wiring diagram that transmits an enormously intricate activity of electric impulses throughout its substance. In the developing brain, young neurons start out from the center and must be guided to their final destinations by specialized adhesion molecules. This process may be akin to traffic lights directing traffic over a very large area like a state. The adhesion molecules signal the billions of neurons to migrate in the right directions toward very specific destinations. This migration is largely completed at birth. Abnormal migration of neurons, in which neurons end up in wrong locations, thus failing to receive appropriate inputs from incoming axons, may result in neurological problems and so-called mental illnesses.

Once the neurons are in the proper location, their next task is to hook up by forming synapses with other neurons, resulting in the wiring diagram of the brain. The neurons must sprout an abundance of axons and dendrites, which must be specifically directed to make contacts with axons and dendrites from a multiplicity of fellow neurons in specific structures; the synapses are sort of miniature organic electrical sockets. In order for the proper connections to be made, specialized molecules, recognition molecules, direct the axons and dendrites to the locations where they are supposed to meet in order for synapses to be constructed. There is a rich brew of different traffic-directing recognition molecules:

PSA-NCAM, NCAM, APP, integrin, N-cadherin, laminin, tenascin, proteoglycans, heparin-binding growth-associated molecules, glial hyaluronate-binding protein, clusterin, and so on.

All in all, a trillion synapses are produced as required throughout life.

Neurotransmission

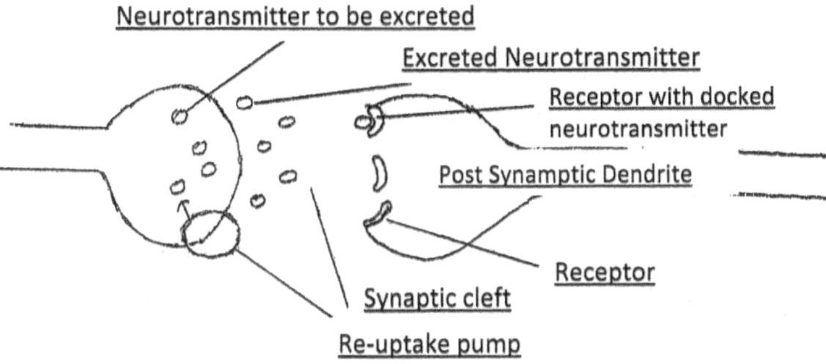

The Synaptic Cleft

The synaptic cleft is at the very end of the axon of the first (pre-synaptic neuron). The end of the axon does not directly make physical contact with the second (post-synaptic neuron) it is communicating with. Instead, it sends out messenger molecules (neurotransmitters) which cross the cleft-space and dock on receptors (which are individualized for different types of them). Once an appropriate neurotransmitter does dock on its receptor (the post synaptic receptor), signal transduction is activated.

The pre-synaptic neuron also has the option of taking back into itself some of the neurotransmitter it has released into the synaptic cleft by means of "re-uptake pumps". The SSRI anti-depressants block the re-uptake pumps, resulting in more neurotransmitter remaining in the synaptic cleft, and therefore more neurotransmitter to dock on post-synaptic receptors.

The Synapse

The neurons collaborate to build the synapses they share with one another. The neurotransmitters that will carry the signal from the first (or presynaptic) neurons are stored in vesicles at the end of their axon terminals. Upon firing, the neurons with the neurotransmitter, in vesicles in the axons, fuses the vesicles with the cell membrane of the axon, discharging the neurotransmitter into the synaptic space, which then diffuses over to the receptors of the receiving neurons that have receptors specific for the particular neurotransmitter, and dock there. If sufficient neurotransmitters have landed on its receptors, the second neuron is induced to fire, continuing the interneuronal communication.

Building a synapse is another precision process. Once the axon has been directed to its proper location, the synapse does not form instantaneously. The collaborating neurons first make a trial contact involving fewer molecules than will be required for the completed synapse. If the trial contact is successful, the molecules are added systematically, in stages, until the synapse is completed. The required components are manufactured after the activation of the specific genes, and they are all transported down the axons and dendrites from the body of the cell. Once a synapse has been constructed, it can be subjected to constant revision and alteration as required. The supplies for construction and maintenance of the synapse include the neurotransmitters, the synaptic vesicles to store them, the receptors, the density molecules, which are needed to give and hold the shape of the synapse, and cellular adhesion molecules to join the structural components of the synapse. In all, a trillion synapses are constructed, and certain neurons may have more than ten thousand.

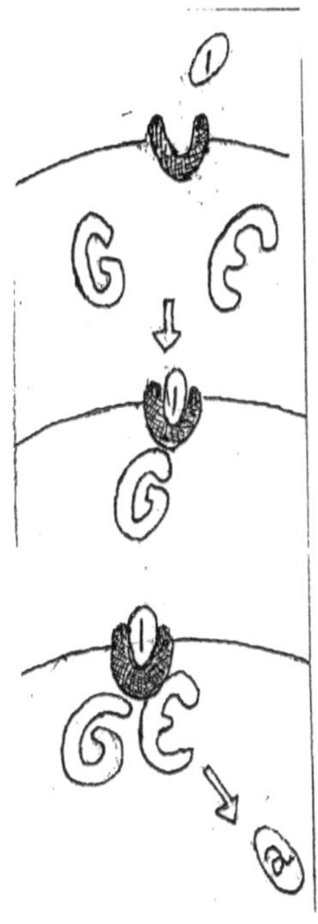

Getting Messages Around The Brain

Conveying messages from outside of neurons, that are from other neurons or from hormones, is like a relay race. The objective is to reach the genes of the receiving neuron to activate them or turn them off. The genes are located in a spherical structure with pores, the nucleolus, in or near the center of the cell in the cytoplasm. There are four distinct communication systems, each with four or more unique different "messenger" molecules. They are named "signal transduction cascades." In the G-protein linked system, illustrated, one of the four systems, the first messenger, 1, docks on the receptor in the outer neuron wall (membrane). When it does so, a protein (G) also joins with the receptor and the first messenger. Next an enzyme (E) also joins the complex, and is triggered to release the second messenger, which finds the third messenger in the cytoplasm, which is then activated, and finds the fourth messenger, which heads towards the nucleolus, through the pores, to position itself on selected genes. The genes can then reverse the entire process, activating messengers to return to the cytoplasm or to influence other neurons.

Glutamate Toxicity

The leading hypothesis for the process leading to the deterioration and destruction of synapses—and in more severe degrees the death of neurons—is glutamate toxicity. Glutamate is an excitatory neurotransmitter widely distributed throughout the brain. During neurological disease states (seizure disorders, brain trauma, ischemic damage to the brain, strokes, multiple sclerosis, amyolateral sclerosis), the brain generates excessive levels of glutamate. But wait! This identical process is operative in the so-called mental disorders: severe recurrent major depression, bipolar disorder, severe OCD, panic disorder, and schizophrenia.[14] Excessive levels of glutamate result in a widening of the openings of calcium channels in the membrane (outer protective skin) of neurons, permitting the buildup of calcium levels inside them. This is toxic to neurons, causing axons and dendrites to deteriorate and also changing the inner organelles in the cytoplasm and genes in the nucleus. At a critical level, apoptosis is triggered, destroying the entire neuron.

In More Detail, Neuronal Communications

The immensity of complexity of the wiring diagram of the brain has been mentioned, but by no means has modern neuroscience been able to chart it in any but rough-hewn outlines. The nitty-gritty details are largely obscure and possibly beyond the reach of science. For example, the precise neuronal connections of every neuron firing during experiences such as listening to and appreciating a symphony or a grand master's painting. Good luck, science! Elaborate chemical and electrical processes are occurring as a key feature of neurotransmission. Abnormal neurotransmission is at the heart of brain diseases—yes, the so-called mental as well as physical diseases.

Signal Transduction

The signaling of the presynaptic neuron to the postsynaptic neuron via the synapse is just like the visible part of an iceberg. On a deeper level, the signal is actually being conveyed from the relevant active genes in the first neuron via a series of messenger molecules through the body of the first neuron to its synapses—and then to the genes of the second neuron by messenger molecules from its receptors in the synapse to its nucleus and often back again in a reversal. This

---

[14] This must be due to mental glutamate causing obscene thoughts, which produce mental toxicity.

extended pathway from the genes of one neuron to another is called the signal transduction pathway.

The brain utilizes a mind-boggling number of neurotransmitters (the communication molecules) that cross the synapse. They can roughly be divided into twelve categories: amines, pituitary peptides, circulating hormones, hypothalamic-releasing hormones, amino acids, gut hormones, opioid peptides, miscellaneous peptides, gases, lipid neurotransmitters, neurokines, tachykinins, and purines. There are at least seventy-five different communicating molecules, but the amine grouping is most relevant for pharmacological treatment since the medications prescribed in psychopharmacology operate on six of these amine neurotransmitters: serotonin, dopamine, norepinephrine/noradrenaline, acetylcholine, glutamate, and gamma-aminobutyric acid.

For treatment purposes, it is essential to understand these important neurotransmitters. They operate in unique circuits, which mediate specific symptoms in neurobiological illnesses (which include so-called mental illnesses!) There are four major signal transduction pathways (cascades) by which they exert their influence: the G protein-linked, ion channel-linked, the nuclear hormone receptors, and the receptor tyrosine kinases. Each begins with a different first messenger.

The following refers to the G protein-linked system in the postsynaptic neuron. Once the first messenger lands on the postsynaptic receptor (of the receiving neuron), a four-part complex is created, which then manufactures the second messenger. The first element of the complex is the neurotransmitter itself, which serves as the first messenger. When it docks on the receptor, it changes the shape of the receptor so that the modified receptor can bind to a G-linked protein in the postsynaptic neuron's cytoplasm (body).

When the third element, the G-linked protein, is attached to the receptor complex, it again changes its shape, which allows the final component, an enzyme in the cytoplasm, to bind to the receptor complex, permitting the bound enzyme to synthesize. The second messenger is then sent off into cytoplasm to find its target, the third messenger in the G-linked system, which then targets a number of different fourth messengers: activated phosphokinase A, DAG (diacylglycerol), activated phosphokinase C, multiple phosphoproteins, and CREB (cyclic AMP response element-binding protein. Similarly, the ion-channel-linked, nuclear hormone system and receptor tyrosine kinase systems each have their own unique first, second, third, and fourth messengers. Having many different signal transduction cascades allows neurons to respond in many diverse ways to a wide array of chemical messaging systems.

The ultimate function of the neurotransmitter-associated signal transduction systems is to regulate and tune gene expression by turning them on or off. All four signal transduction cascades end with the last molecule affecting gene expression. What is important is not just the number of genes activated, but when, how often, and in what sequence the genes are expressed. An important molecule, CREB (CAMP response-element binding protein), functions as a transcription factor by landing on the coding regions of the targeted genes, inducing the genes to be transcribed (copied) by an enzyme, RNA polymerase, resulting in a new RNA molecule, a mirror-image copy of the DNA of the genes that are being duplicated.

Gene expression occurs in two waves. First, early genes are expressed. They activate the promoter regions of late genes, which are the workhorses of eventual protein manufacture that sustain the overall neuron and its function. There are two subtypes of early genes, C Fos and C Jun, which when activated, produce their respective proteins, Fos and Jun, which can be considered fifth messengers. Fos and Jun combine to make the Fos-Jun combination protein, which acts as the sixth messenger transcription factor for late genes.

The product of late genes can be any protein the neuron needs, such as an enzyme, transport factors, growth factors, and other vital proteins. One specific example of the entire sequence of gene expression is the receptor life cycle. The genes, which when activated, code for the manufacture of receptors for a given neurotransmitter is transcribed into RNA, which leaves the nucleus and travels to the ribosomes in the cell body where the RNA is translated into partially formed receptor proteins that travel the Golgi apparatus (an organelle) where transformation into the final receptor proteins occurs.

The completed receptor proteins are placed in vesicles for transport to the cell membrane to form the actual receptor. When the specific neurotransmitter it is meant to receive docks on the receptor (the first messenger), it manufactures and then sends off the second messenger, which eventually transmits the signal back to the nucleus as previously described. When the genes determine there are an excessive number of receptors for a specific neurotransmitter, the membrane to which the receptor is attached will indent and form a pit that breaks off as a vesicle to transport the superfluous receptor to a lysosome in the cytoplasm, which destroys it. There is an ongoing dynamic process of receptor manufacture and destruction, depending on the neuron requirements.

The neuron, by regulating its gene expression, produces all the parts required for survival and optimal functioning: synaptogenesis, neurogenesis, apoptosis, manufacture of enzymes, growth factors, and other vital proteins. A vast number of neurons, functioning conjointly, result in the human capacities for learning, remembering, and purposeful behavior—the entire realm of human experience. Unfortunately, irregularities of gene expression and correlated neuronal dysfunctions result in symptoms of serious brain illnesses. Because such dysfunctions are basic to the so-called mental illnesses—as they are for neurological disorders—how can there be any rationale for maintaining the treacherous dichotomy? Who benefits from this dichotomy? Who suffers?

CHAPTER 7A

The Mental Health Care System

The purpose of any effective health care system should be to anticipate the vulnerability to the onset of a given disease, institute measures to prevent the onset (primary prevention), institute diagnostic and treatment measures on a timely basis at the earliest stage of the disease (secondary prevention), and minimize symptoms and disability throughout the course of the disease (tertiary prevention). In general, all the medical specialties from allergy and anesthesiology to urology and wilderness medicine achieve these purposes. Only the so-called mental health care system, cut off from all the other medical specialties and malfunctioning in splendid isolation, fails spectacularly.

Henry A. Nasrallah, MD, in an editorial in *Current Psychiatry* (November 2013), has a profound appreciation for the human brain, a glorious organ. He considers it is in a position of supremacy above all the body's other organs because it is the source of our transcendent minds. Through its mental functions, our most distinct human abilities are manifested: self-awareness, thinking, speaking, remembering, communicating, and deciding.

He does have a bone to pick at the shades of ignorance, especially surrounding the mind and its mental disorders, particularly at prominent individuals who trumpet their ignorance and misconceptions, feeding the negative stereotyping of the disorders and its practitioners.

He comments about David Brooks, a *New York Times* columnist whose pronouncements on mental illness makes Nasrallah's heart sink:

> Earlier in the year (2014), this influential individual boldly declared that psychiatry is not a real science, that the psychiatric diagnostic manual DSM-5 warranted disparagement, and that psychiatrists are heroes of uncertainty.

Dr. Nasrallah's disappointment escalated into alarm when he considered Brooks had millions of readers who regard him as credible, and in whom ugly misconceptions, virulent falsehoods, and malicious propaganda about psychiatry would deter people from seeking the help they need.

Nasrallah extols the colossal body of scientific evidence that informs psychiatry and the biological basis for the mental illnesses, and he acknowledges that psychiatrists, by failing to disseminate the neuroanatomic, neurophysiologic, neurochemical, and molecular underpinnings of the perceptual, affective thought and behavioral symptoms of these illnesses are partly to blame.

Nasrallah does not pursue the question of blame to its ultimate conclusion. The so-called specialty of psychiatry is dominated by therapists (therapy psychiatrists) who have a powerful incentive to underplay these biological underpinnings, firstly because they are resistant to undertaking the huge task of understanding in detail the multiplicity of biological mechanisms associated with these illnesses, and secondly, because their bread is buttered by their practices in which their chief source of income is the so-called weekly psychodynamic forty-five-minute therapy session for each of their patients.

The public is completely uninformed about the variations in psychiatric practice. How can those with the more serious, symptomatic, disabling so-called mental illnesses know that they need to seek diagnostic evaluation and ongoing medical (psychopharmacological) treatment from that small minority of psychiatrists who are physicians first (brain psychiatrists), who expend considerable time and energy mastering the brain mechanisms that cause the so-called mental illnesses, and the corresponding psychopharmacological treatments that manipulate their symptoms in a favorable direction.

This is not to say psychotherapy is not a useful treatment for some so-called mental disorders. There are, however, a great many lay therapists, MSWs, and PhDs who are more proficient than psychiatrists in administering specialized therapies such as cognitive and behavioral ones for which psychiatrists generally do not have specialized training or expertise. As we shall see, the true medical specialty of neurology, the other specialty that concentrates on the brain, also employs psychosocial interventions in the form of physical therapy and rehabilitative therapies, but it appropriately arranges for the physician, the neurologist, to first utilize diagnostic and therapeutic medical expertise to evaluate the patient and their brain and then referring, if indicated, for the adjunctive therapies. This is much safer for the patients of neurologists since the physical ailments of the brain are diagnosed and medically treated up front rather than being missed, ignored, inaccurately diagnosed, and brain treatment not administered at all or deferred as occurs in the mental health care system. Most prospective patients are seen by nonmedical therapists or therapy psychiatrists before, if they even get to, highly trained psychiatric physicians (brain psychiatrists) who voluntarily submerge themselves in neuroscience and sophisticated complex pharmacological treatments.

The Morbidity and Mortality Associated with So-Called Mental Illnesses

In 2015, a large-scale systematic review and analysis to investigate in detail the burden of these illnesses was completed ("Mortality in Mental Disorders and Global Disease Burden Implications: A Systematic Review and Meta-Analysis," Elizabeth R. Walker, PhD,

MPH, MAT, Robin E. McGee, MPH, Benjamin G. Druss, MD, MPH.)[15] Previously, a number of scientific studies had illustrated the increases in mortality due to so-called mental illnesses, including psychotic disorders, major depressive disorders, bipolar disorder, and anxiety disorders, in comparison to individuals not having these disorders. The objective of this study was to conduct the widest survey ever undertaken to further examine the link. They reviewed all the relevant studies, a total of 2,481, and selected the best from a methodological and scientific standard, leaving 203 derived from twenty-nine countries across six continents. The all-cause mortality of individuals having mental disorders was nearly two and a half times greater than comparison individuals without mental disorders. The total deaths in the former was 338,381. The largest category of deaths in all-cause mortality was from natural causes (67.3 percent). This group included most of the chronic medical diseases, cardiovascular, metabolic, and neurological, i.e. heart disease, diabetes, stroke, etc., and 17 percent fell into the unnatural causes portion (deaths attributable to accidents, poverty, insufficient preventive services, lower-quality medical care, and suicide). It was determined individuals with so-called mental disorders lose more than ten years of life in comparison to individuals without mental illnesses. Although longevity is increasing in the latter, those in the former are not participating. It is necessary to emphasize the vast proportion of premature deaths among the so-called mentally ill are not due to suicide. The scientific data firmly establishes that these so-called mental disorders culminate in significant increases in physical mortality burden.

In addition to severe mental symptoms, disrupted life desires and goals, and restricting, defeating disabilities, the mentally ill are also being afflicted with severe general medical illnesses more than other individuals. They are experiencing a degradation of their time alive by more than ten years. What kind of services and treatments are available to help them and reduce the sum total of illness, loss, pain, and humiliation they contend with?

---

[15] *JAMA Psychiatry*, 2015 April 72 (14): 334-341.

Representative Tim Murphy of the Eighteenth District of Pennsylvania has extensively studied the mental health care system. He also has had a doctorate in psychology for thirty years. At the behest of Congress, he undertook a nationwide evaluation of mental health care, visiting many communities over a year and a half. His preliminary pronouncement of what he learned was profound shock at the fragmentation and inadequacies, which he could only label "archaic." Of the approximately ten million people with the most severe mental illnesses, 40 percent were not receiving care. He noted many barriers to timely care. He received thousands of letters, calls, and emails from families describing the impossible hurdles faced by them in finding appropriate, effective help for loved ones, and by extension, how there were also ripple effects in their communities. Among the manifold obstacles: an insufficiency of unqualified providers, the stigma associated with mental illness (in spite of goodly sums of federal tax dollars to reduce stigma), legal barriers to care, including HIPPA state laws that cut off communications about an ill adult loved one from their families, the role of legal advocates and the anti-psychiatry activists who see their mission as preserving the liberty of the very severely mentally ill, who as a result, instead of receiving needed treatment, are funneled into jails or the streets. The police are usually the first responders when mentally ill individuals are causing a disturbance, but if providers most of whom are not even physicians, let alone brain psychiatrists).

In the *Journal of Current Psychiatry,* Nasrallah expresses his frustration at how society is indifferent to the suffering of the mentally ill.[16] He describes anosognosia as a neurological symptom in which patients can have symptoms but are absolutely convinced they do not have the symptom. This can occur in strokes in which a patient is paralyzed to some degree—for example, an arm—but deny it. Similarly, the mentally ill are obviously suffering in society, but society

---

[16] Nasrallah, Henry A. "The Scourge of Societal Anosognosia About the Mentally Ill," *Current Psychiatry,* June 15, 2016 (6): 19, 23–24.

does not see it and is indifferent to it. The exact opposite is true for physical disease.

The Center for Disease Control in May 2016 released information that the suicide rate increased by 24 percent between 1999 and 2014. This fact got only casual mention and was soon forgotten. If there had been a similar increase in heart disease or cancer, there would be a public outcry followed by demands by Congress, the National Institutes of Health, and the Center for Disease Control to address such a catastrophic rise by directing billions of dollars of additional spending for prevention.

Mental illness also has deadly consequences. In 2014, 42,773 people died by suicide, and hundreds of thousands were injured and maimed in suicide attempts. Tens of millions suffer from depression, bipolar disorder, schizophrenia, anxiety disorders, post-traumatic stress disorder, and substance abuse disorders and may never receive timely treatment that could save their lives or reduce their suffering and disabilities. Nasrallah lists a number of hazards the mentally ill endure because of society's anosognosia associated with mental illness. There is a lack of compassion in contrast to sympathy expressed toward people with medical ailments like cardiovascular disease or cancer. Society continues to portray mental illnesses as resulting from character flaws, personal weakness, or failure in contrast to those with physical diseases like Parkinson's disease or multiple sclerosis. Society permits the stigmatization and its attendant humiliation of the mentally ill to continue unabated. There is widespread discrimination against the mentally ill by insurance companies in spite of parity laws, but society turns a blind eye. In association with restrictions of health coverage, there is much lower use of lifesaving diagnostic and treatment procedures available to those patients, compared to the non-mentally ill. There is an associated indifference to the drastic increase in mortality; if they are not acutely suicidal or homicidal, they are quickly returned to the community.

As a result of mental illness, some individuals may not understand they need treatment, so they are just left to their own (inadequate) devices. Representative Murphy notes that in no other medical discipline is this allowed to occur; if an individual has a stroke and can't ask for care, they are nevertheless taken to an appropriate treatment center. In other words, the mental health care system does not act to prevent a crisis; it only picks up the pieces after a crisis. In the meantime, Murphy notes that severe mental illnesses are actually brain illnesses, and by the time any help is received, the brain has been damaged, progressive deterioration is occurring, and the subjects are afflicted with permanent disabilities. A great many end up incarcerated or homeless. He labels this inhumane. He put a great deal of effort into overhauling the mental health care system as reflected in the Helping Families in Mental Health Crisis Act (HR 3717) from 2013. The bill is meant to refocus care and resources on the more severely ill, integrate mental and physical care, modify state and HIPPA laws to facilitate communications, and incentivize communities to apply modern treatment approaches. At the end of 2016, it still resides in committees.

Representative Murphy notes the particular pain inflicted on patients who are so enveloped in despair that suicide seems more merciful than continued existence (agonizing symptoms, lost dreams, and the injuries of losses). So many people—out of ignorance, prejudice, or deficiencies of compassion—secretly think of them as heathens or cowardly or selfish. He had heard those very expressions when some individuals were referring to Robin Williams. He concluded these insults demonstrate that, even after the expenditure of millions of dollars to attenuate stigma through public awareness campaigns about the causes of suicide, stigma remains pervasive.

He feels it is critical to dispel common misconceptions about suicide and elaborate on what he characterizes as myths about it. The first myth is suicide is very uncommon, but in reality, more than 1.3 million people annually have serious suicide attempts, and 40,000 die by suicide. The second myth is those who die by suicide should have just pulled it together and carried on. He clarifies over 90 percent of suicides occur in the midst of a serious mental illness, such as schizophrenia, bipolar disorder, or major depression. He notes depression increases suicide risk by 50 percent. Mental illnesses can fundamentally change the pathways of the brain, making it difficult for those without these diseases to comprehend what compels an individual to take his or her own life.

Furthermore, some who die by suicide believe their disappearance eases the burden on their families. A third myth is that suicide is a well-planned, thoughtful act. Most who commit suicide do it impulsively in response to powerful emotional pain. At least 70 percent of suicides are triggered by intense distress in the span of five to sixty minutes.

He summarizes again how these myths persist in spite of public awareness campaigns that have failed to educate and reduce stigma. Suicide rates have not been significantly reduced among younger people, and the rate has increased 28 percent among those aged thirty-five to sixty-four. Suicide by suffocation or hanging has increased 81 percent. He exclaims too many lives are at stake to allow the current situation to be perpetuated.

Miriam, a thirty-four-year-old dental technician from Connecticut, died after Washington police shot her in her car. An eighteen-month-old child, believed to be her daughter, was taken to the hospital and found to be unharmed. Miriam had led the police on a wild chase from the White House to the Capitol. The chase created panic in the Capitol, and members of Congress were ordered to stay in place. A swarm of police descended on the scene after she struck a security fence outside the White House and hit a security service officer. Sources subsequently disclosed her history of mental health problems. The dentist for whom she previously worked fired her in 2012 after patients complained she was too rough with them. The dentist noted she had seemed increasingly distressed after an unwanted pregnancy. The police concluded she may have believed Obama was stalking her. A relative said she may have suffered from postpartum depression.

More than a year and a half passed between the time of her initial symptoms, when the dentist fired her, until her death. Was her illness ever recognized? Did she have an opportunity to receive treatment that could have saved her life? Did anyone notice her symptoms, particularly since she was the mother of an infant? Obamacare has produced a noticeable increase in the mental health care availability of uninsured low-income Americans. In the states that have expanded Medicaid, the federal government provides full reimbursement for treatment. An estimated 350,000 people received treatment in 2014. In the other states, 568,000 individuals with diagnosed serious mental illness did not. In Florida and Texas, 66,723 and 62,400 respectively were left to their own devices. It is estimated a third of the inmates in jails across the country have severe, untreated mental illness. After they serve their sentences, they are returned to their communities in which they account for a third of the homeless who eventually circulate back to hospital ERs or jails.

The so-called mental health care system requires an even more drastic overhaul than Representative Murphy suggests. The term *mental illness* and all the associated toxic stigmatizing thinking conjured up by that frame of reference must be extinguished from our thoughts, brains, and minds.

GLOSSARY

basal ganglia. A group of subcortical nuclei responsible primarily for motor control, among other roles.

catecholamines. Another name for a neurotransmitter grouping including dopamine, norepinephrine, and epinephrine.

catecholaminergic systems. Refers to neurotransmitters associated with the stress response.

caudate nucleus (also called striatum. A paired subcortical structure associated with basal ganglia involved in memory and learning.

cerebellum. A region at the posterior part of the brain important for coordination of movement.

corpus callosum. Connects the right and left hemispheres of the brain. A large band of nerve fibers.

dendritic spine. A small membranous protrusion from a neuron's dendrite, receiving input from axon of another neuron.

frontal cortex. One of the four major lobes of the cerebral cortex located at the front of the brain.

hippocampus. The part of the brain involved in memory formation and memory storage. It is part of the limbic system.

middle prefrontal cortex. The part of the prefrontal cortex that mediates decision-making. It's located behind the forehead.

neurotransmitter transporter (reuptake pump). The transport of previously secreted neurotransmitters back into the neuron.

parietal cortex. One of the four major lobes. Its main responsibility is processing sensory information.

plasticity. The capacity to adopt by essential brain components, i.e., continuous alteration of neurons, neuropathways, and synapses to meet the brain's needs. Neurotransmitters are released from the presynaptic neuron, many of which will land on its specific receptors on the receiving neuron. Receptors are large proteins that initiate the transduction cascades.

reuptake pump. See neurotransmitter transporters.

single nucleotide polymorphisms (SNPs). A variation in a single nucleotide that occurs at a specific position in the genome. Nucleotides are organic molecules that serve as the building blocks of DNA and RNA, the molecules of heredity. (See illustration).

synaptic cleft. A tiny opening between neurons that neurotransmitters traverse from one neuron to another.

synaptic transmission. The process of a neurotransmitter crossing from one neuron to the next via the synaptic cleft to transmit a signal.

This nucleotide contains the five-carbon sugar deoxyribose, a nitrogenous base called adenine, and one phosphate group. Together, the deoxyribose and adenine make up a nucleoside (specifically, a deoxyribonucleoside) called deoxyadenosine. With the one phosphate group included, the whole structure is considered a deoxyribonucleotide (a nucleotide constituent of DNA) with the name deoxyadenosine monophosphate.

Genetic Transmission

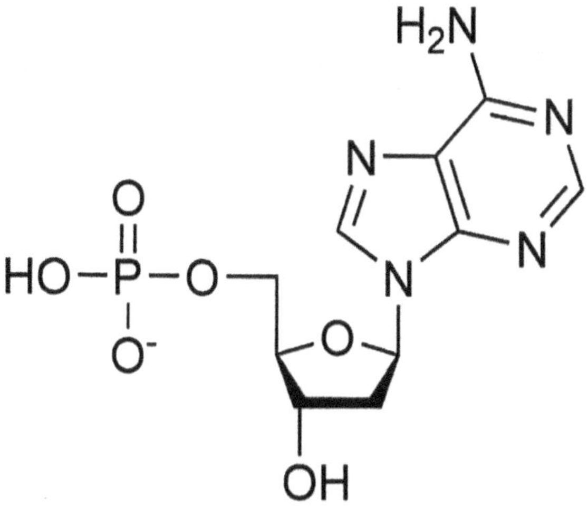

The nucleotide molecule: turning the fertilized egg into billions of neurons

CHAPTER 8

ADHD

Prepare yourself to learn how deep unconscious conflict causes ADHD. Therapy psychiatrist theoreticians have deciphered that collisions between the id and the superego occurring at a rate of seven per minute cause such distraction that the individuals with ADHD cannot focus their attention and are put into a state of hyperarousal in which they cannot sit still or remain calm and quiet for normal periods of time.

The past several decades of neuroscientific research in genetics, molecular biology, and neuroimaging have confirmed this illness has a neurobiological basis.[17] Genes for the dopamine (DA) and norepinephrine (NE) neurotransmitter systems have been studied. Abnormal single nucleotide polymorphisms (SNPs) and variable repeated sequences of nucleotides affect the DA receptor D4 (DRD4), the DA receptor D5 (DRD5), DA transporter (SLC6A3/DAT1, serotonin receptor 1B (HTR1B), serotonin transporter (SLC6A4/5HTT), and synaptosomal-associated protein (SNAP-25) genes. The specific genes are in parentheses.

There is further evidence from the analysis of high-ranking SNPs associated with basic biological "processes" such as brain development,

---

[17] *Pediatric Research* (2011) 69, 69R-76R; soi:10.1203/PDR.obo13e318212b4of. Neurobiology of Attention Deficit/Hyperactivity Disorder. Diane Purper-Ouakil, Nicolas Ramoz, et al.

maturation, neuronal migration, plasticity, and genetic dysfunctions in ADHD. Genes influencing the volumes of critical brain structures like the prefrontal cortex and the caudate nucleus have been implicated. Also, varieties of genes have been determined to be involved in the formation of abnormal protein complexes, modifications of neuronal structures, changes in dendritic spine morphology (shape), and abnormal synaptic transmission.

Catecholaminergic systems have been studied since they are the main targets of the medications used to alleviate the symptoms of ADHD. Most of the medications increase the availability of catecholamines in the synaptic cleft. All the stimulant medications optimize catecholamine signaling in the prefrontal cortex by blocking DA and NE transporters (reuptake pumps) and enhancing the release of the neurotransmitters. They also inhibit an enzyme, monoamine oxidase, that metabolizes the neurotransmitters. It is thought DA stimulation has therapeutic effects by the weakening of inappropriate network connections (producing a decrease of noise.) Enhanced NE transmission may function by strengthening appropriate connections, producing an increase in normal signaling.

Neuroimaging studies have identified a number of brain regions implicated in ADHD: the frontal and parietal cortex, basal ganglia, cerebellum, hippocampus, and corpus callosum. A detailed review of neural networks in these structures indicates diffuse and also more specific alterations involving decreased connectivity, particularly in a permanent circuit, the striatal-partial-cerebellum. Interestingly, stimulant treatment improves connectivity.

White matter tracts in the brain also show evidence of dysfunctions in anatomical connections. Longitudinal studies (in which patients have neuroimaging studies over a period of years) have demonstrated delayed maturation of the middle prefrontal cortex, parietal cortex, and hippocampus. In some instances, patients also experience progressive volume loss associated with persistence of or worsening of symptoms. On the other hand, normalization of volumes is associated with symptomatic improvement.

In an educational article, "What is Attention Deficit Hyperactivity Disorder,"[18] it is recommended the family of an affected child talk with a mental health specialist with experience in childhood mental disorders such as ADHD. If the pediatrician wants to refer for treatment rather than treating the child him/herself, there is no mention of who or what type of mental health professional should be utilized and not even a hint that it should be a specialized medical professional. Since psychiatry labels ADHD as just a mental problem, why would any specialized medical provider even need to be considered? All that's required is any type of mental health therapist.

ADHD is a neurobiological illness—and not a mental problem. Epilepsy is another neurobiological illness. The neurologist is the first professional to evaluate the patient.

Expertise is required—not dangerous, inappropriate half measures—but the competence of a brain psychiatrist learned in the brain mechanism and skilled in the pharmacological treatment of the illness. That is the equivalent of the neurologist who does the brain first and then draws in adjunctive professionals.

To do an adequate job of diagnosing and treating ADHD, specialized medical expertise is necessary. ADHD is not an easy diagnosis to make or simple to treat. Physicians in all medical specialties—from allergy to urology, with the sole exception of therapy psychiatrists—are rigorously trained in making a differential diagnosis. They think of all possible diseases and circumstances that could explain the symptoms the patient has presented with before making the final diagnoses. Making a differential diagnosis requires a disciplined, structured approach rather than the structureless ambling interviewing approach of the therapy psychiatrist. A careful history must be taken, the presence of all relevant symptoms and diseases cataloged, and data solicited from other sources of information, family, spouse, and in the case of school-aged children, input from academic settings. Then comes the exercise of making a differential diagnosis (after supplementation with the results of laboratory tests that have

18 The National Institute of Mental Health: www.nimh.nih.gov

been ordered on the basis of a provisional differential diagnosis) and a physical examination.

ADHD can be simulated by other conditions. Expertise is required to distinguish it from fool's gold. Some children have emotional or disciplinary problems that can be erroneously attributed to ADHD. Most children get distracted, act impulsively, or struggle to concentrate at times. Since these are also key symptoms of ADHD, distinctions must be made. Are these excessive, long-term, continuous behaviors that affect all aspects of the child's life? Are these more severe when compared to their peers? Do they occur in several settings rather than in one place? Even a child with ADHD can control their behaviors in some settings if they are getting individual attention or are free to focus on enjoyable activities.

Learning disabilities can simulate ADHD, and so can other psychiatric syndromes, oppositional defiant disorder, conduct disorder, and Tourette Syndrome. Contrary to the treacherous dichotomy, there is no easily visible boundary between the psychiatrists' mental illness of ADHD and physical illnesses such as undetected seizures, middle ear infections causing hearing problems, visual problems, or systemic medical illnesses.

For pharmacological treatments, all you need is a prescription pad and a pen. Just write the name of any old drug at whatever dosage and then forget about it. Take two aspirins, and you'll be okay in the morning.

Even though it is counterintuitive, stimulants should improve the symptoms of ADHD. Numerous scientific studies have confirmed they reduce hyperactivity and impulsivity, improve the ability to focus, and facilitate learning and job performance. Interestingly, they may improve physical coordination. There is no cookie-cutter formula that the same medication and dosage will work for most children. There are at least seventeen branded formulations of stimulants. In many cases, the prescriber must be experienced enough to select the most appropriate preparation for a given patient and then titrate it carefully to minimize side effects while reaching the most effective dosage.

This is critical for the patient whose success in academics, work, and relationships can be riding on the pharmacological expertise of the prescriber. A one-size-fits-all approach will backfire, and the prescribers' insensitivity or inexperience regarding side effects can permanently discourage patients, condemning them to a suboptimal life trajectory.

Unfortunately, inexperienced prescribers (some pediatricians and many therapy psychiatrists) may prescribe an antipsychotic, selectively focusing on behavioral disturbances and missing the diagnosis of ADHD. Others lack the capacity to differentiate ADHD from childhood-adolescent bipolar disorder, precipitating manic or psychotic episodes, suicide attempts, and hospitalizations by not prescribing a mood stabilizer before starting a stimulant medication. Also, ADHD many remain undiagnosed until later in life and be a source of cognitive disturbance and disability. The internist or therapy psychiatrist most likely will never think of that possibility.

Another detail patients should be aware of in making an accurate diagnosis of ADHD is rather tedious. The provider should carefully complete a rather long symptom checklist as well as having parents and teachers supply sufficient information.

Many providers short-circuit this rather lengthy process by going on a hunch. That is much quicker!

GLOSSARY

amygdala. A bilateral set of neurons linked to fear and pleasure response.

cingulate cortex, anterior part. The frontal part of the frontal cortex region plays a role in motivational functions, decision-making, and outcome monitoring.

GABA (gamma-aminobutyric acid). An amino acid that acts to inhibit transmission of nerve impulses and counters glutamate.

HPA axis (hypothalamic pituitary axis). Directly affects the functions of the thyroid, adrenal glands, and gonads. Plays a central role in stress response.

hypothalamus. A part of the brain that produces many hormones that control other hormones in the body.

limbic system subdivisions. Insular cortex, cingulate cortex, hippocampus, and amygdalae.

medulla. Plays a major role in controlling many of the automated functions of the midbrain. Associated with vision, hearing, sleep/wake, arousal (alertness), and temperature regulation.

neuropeptide. Small protein molecules that can act like neurotransmitters.

occipital cortex. One of the four major lobes located at the back of the brain, serves as primary visual cortex.

parietal lobe, left interior part. Body image, visual spatial perception, language, consciousness.

serotonin 5-HT1A receptors. A subtype of serotonin receptor that may help antidepressant drugs have benefit.

thalamus. Relays sensory impulses from body to the cortex and is active in perception.

CHAPTER 9

Anxiety Disorders

In *The Diagnostic and Statistical Manual of Mental Disorders* published by the American Psychiatric Association, a number of anxiety disorders are listed along with multiple diagnostic criteria. To get to what is important, however, the author will discuss panic disorder. The word *anxiety* does not appear to be portraying something to be overly concerned about. Everybody experiences anxiety—so what? Think positive! Go about your business! It's just a mental thing!

Individuals with severe panic disorder sometimes appear to be severely symptomatic. They monopolize medical resources, for example, often presenting at emergency rooms as if they are having a real medical crisis, having exaggerated fears they are having a heart attack or stroke. In this fashion, expensive diagnostic tests, electrocardiograms, multiple laboratory blood tests, even CAT scans and expensive consultations with a cardiologist or neurologist are ordered out of medical-legal anxieties a real physical diagnosis will be missed, leaving an opening for malpractice attorneys to enter the picture. And as all this unnecessary (from a purely medical perspective) activity is occurring, a patient with an actual heart attack or stroke may be left waiting in the hall.

Characteristic of panic disorder are recurrent, unexpected panic attacks. There can be a variety of symptoms which come out of the blue for no apparent reason. These include heart palpitations, speeded heartbeat, sweating, trembling, chest pain, nausea, abdominal pain, dizziness, feeling faint, chills, heat sensations, numbness, fear of going crazy, even fear of dying. Really, now, shouldn't an individual experiencing these symptoms realize they're just emotional, just mental, and calm themselves down?

Another symptom is a sensation of shortness of breath, which can manifest as air being cut off, complete smothering, which at its most intense is associated with an emotional terror. Any individual who has experienced such suffocation will tell you it certainly felt absolutely real to them. Are they lying or exaggerating to win pampering or sympathy? That brings up the discussion of waterboarding. Individuals who are waterboarded are not physically injured or mutilated. Fingers are not cut off, and no bones are broken.

During a waterboarding session, which generally lasts about twenty minutes (unlike severe, repetitive panic attacks, which can last a day or several days), the subject is restrained on his back but otherwise not deliberately physically injured. Cloth or cellophane is placed over the breathing passages, and water is continuously poured onto the face from a distance of twelve to twenty-four inches. The end result is the victim experiences a sensation of suffocation by drowning. It is the intensity of the experience of suffocating that inflicts the most distress. CIA officers who have subjected themselves to the technique have lasted an average of fourteen seconds before capitulating.[19] The technique, which has been utilized since the Spanish Inquisition, is a preferred method of torture since it produces no marks upon the body. Dr. Allen Keller, the director of the Bellevue Hospital/New York University Program for Survivors of Torture [20]reports victims are traumatized years later—as are many patients with severe, recurrent panic disorder, in which the illness is never diagnosed to begin with or is inadequately treated.

Anxiety disorders, like mood disorders, are characterized by a complex interplay between neuroendocrine, neurotransmitter,

---

[19] Waterboarding. From Wikipedia.

[20] Ibid.

and neuroanatomical disruptions. There is a high degree of interconnectivity between the neurotransmitter and neuropeptide-containing circuits in the brain stem, limbic areas, and the cerebral cortex. Identifying the most functionally relevant dysfunctions associated with the major anxiety disorders (panic disorder, post-traumatic stress disorder, and generalized anxiety disorder) is a matter of some complexity. Nevertheless, neuroscience has made much progress.

Frontal cortical regions regulate emotions and impulses via messaging to the emotional-processing regions, thereby exerting behavioral control. The prefrontal frontal cortex subdivision is responsible for planning, decision-making, weighing the potential consequences of behaviors, and assessing the appropriateness of social responses. The orbito-frontal cortex controls impulses, regulates mood, and classifies incoming information. The ventromedial subdivision regulates reward processing and additional aspects of emotional response. The emotional processing brain structures, generally referred to as the limbic system, are also subdivided into the insular cortex, cingulate cortex, hippocampus, and amygdalae.

The hippocampus can be directly impacted by severe anxiety symptoms, causing it to lose volume via neuron injury or apoptosis and inhibition of neurogenesis (the birth of new neurons). It has a number of responsibilities, particularly controlling and regulating the stress response of the hypothalamic-pituitary-adrenal axis (HPA), which if not modulated, secretes excess cortisol, damaging neuronal structures and functions. The amygdalae process emotionally relevant incoming stimuli and initiate the corresponding behavioral responses. They are also intimately associated with the expression of fear and the triggering of defensive behavior. They are heavily connected to multiple brain areas: cortical regions, hippocampus, thalamus, and hypothalamus.

The communication within and between each brain region utilizes a host of different molecules, including the major neurotransmitters, serotonin, norepinephrine, dopamine, gamma-aminobutyric acid, glutamate, and acetylcholine, but they are but the tip of the iceberg. Additional communicating molecules include vesicular monoamine transporters, vasopressin, oxytocin, SERT, neurotonin dopamine transporter, MAOI, COMT, neuropeptides, CCK, galanin, NPY, AVP, CRF, and CCK.

Each anxiety disorder also has genetic and environmental causes. In summary, it should be obvious multiple etiological factors are operating synergistically, which accounts for symptomatology. If it were only so simple as the therapy psychiatrists believe, that deep unconscious conflicts in the id, if combated by penetrating incisive, pinpoint psychodynamic interpretations will relieve the symptoms of anxiety disorders.

More on Panic Disorder

Maybe it is that simple. If you open up a skull of a recently deceased person with panic disorder, the brain tissue looks fine to the naked eye. Perhaps all this neuroscience chemical stuff is nonsense! The brain looks fine. There is no obvious injury. That should decide the issue—panic disorder is a mental problem! There is no evidence of a physical problem, no bruising, no tears or rips, and no missing pieces!

Actually, the biological dysfunctions underlying panic disorder are multifaceted and intricate, involving an interplay of alterations in brain tissue, metabolism, neurotransmitter and neuroendocrine signaling, receptor functioning, systems governing vulnerability to stress, particularly the HPA axis (hypothalamic-pituitary axis), and genes.

Neuroimaging studies have revealed a number of alterations: neuroanatomical, metabolic, in blood supply distribution, and concentrations of neurotransmitters and neuropeptides. There is reduced metabolism in the left inferior parietal lobe. Paradoxically, the uptake of glucose is increased in the amygdala, hippocampus, thalamus, midbrain, medulla, and cerebellum. There is an overall reduction in blood flow to both cerebral cortices and an asymmetry.

Certain localities, the right medial and superior lobes, have a paradoxical increase in flow. The hippocampus and amygdala have a noticeable reduction in flow, except during a panic attack, when there is a dramatic increase in the right amygdala.

There are distinct differences (from healthy individuals) in the concentrations of neurotransmitters, neuropeptides, and receptors. There is a lower baseline concentration of GABA (gamma-aminobutyric acid) in several brain areas, the occipital cortex, the ACC (anterior cingulate cortex), and the basal ganglia. There is decreased benzodiazine binding in the left hippocampus (signifying a deficiency of receptors for binding calming neurotransmitters) and decreased binding to 5-HT1A receptors, likewise signifying deficiencies in down-regulating excitatory anxiety. The 5-HT1A receptor has wide distribution in the midbrain, bilateral temporal lobes, and the thalamus. There are concomitant increased levels of the excitatory neurotransmitter glutamate. Noradrenaline concentrations likewise are increased. In panic disorder, the circuits transmitting it are altered.

CCK is a neuropeptide, which if given to healthy volunteers, will induce panic attacks. It is hypothesized in panic disorder there may be an excess of CCK receptors responding to endogenous (made in the body) CCK. All six of the major monoamine neurotransmitters are accompanied by neuropeptides, at least sixteen in all, adding to the complexity of potential biological dysregulations.

The HPA axis has been mentioned. A number of inputs may make it hypersensitive in panic disorder. The HPA is an important regulator of the stress response, which if unregulated, will trigger exaggerated, involuntary stress emotions.

Panic disorder is the most heritable of the anxiety disorders. First-degree relations of a patient with panic disorder have a sevenfold greater risk of also developing it. There have been a number of studies linking panic disorder to sets of genes, particularly on chromosomes 2g and 15g. These genetic associations are complex. As an example, genes for panic disorder are found in association with important receptors, neurotransmitters, neuropeptides, and others, such as COMT, adenosine 2A receptor, CCK, CCK receptor B, 5-HT2A receptor, and monoamine oxidase-A.

<u>The Hypothalamic – Pituitary – Adrenal Axis</u>

The hypothalamus, an area in the lower brain, manages much of the behavior of hormones, which play a wide role in the brain and the body. It secretes corticotropin releasing hormone (CRH) which activates the anterior pituitary gland, in turn to secrete adrenocortitropin the adrenal gland via the bloodstream, stimulating the release of cortisol, which while exerting it's effects on the body, also supplies negative feedback to the hypothalamus.

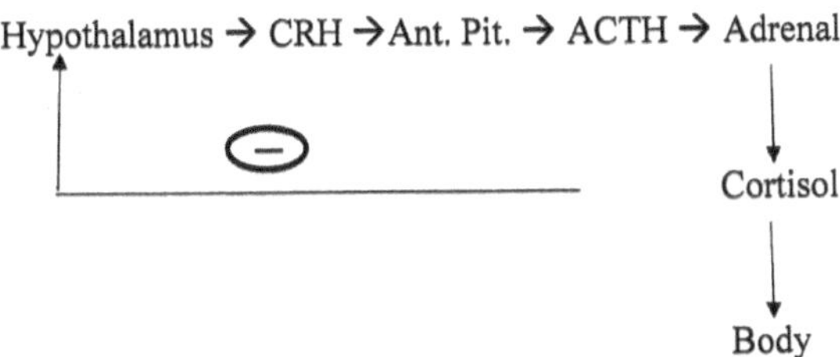

Social Anxiety Disorder

Individuals with this anxiety disorder become markedly anxious and uncomfortable in social situations. Often, they will avoid such situations, for example, declining invitations or avoiding conversation. They are acutely concerned that their anxiety will be observed by others or they will somehow come across the wrong way during introductions and conversations, resulting in humiliation, embarrassment, or rejection. Now, surely, this is a mental problem that is easy to overcome—just relax, smile, put on a pretty or handsome face, and be friendly. Stop being foolish and loosen up!

Interestingly, however, as with panic disorder (as well as PTSD and generalized anxiety disorder), hyperactivity of the amygdalae and associated limbic areas is a central finding. Symptom severity is directly proportional to the degree of bilateral amygdala activation, and it reverses with successful treatment. Rather than going through a narration again of the multiplicity of biological processes and mechanisms causative of social anxiety disorder, we'll just list them: (Warning—read this at your peril!)

Subcortical, limbic, paralimbic activity increased; autonomic emotional processing increased; decreased activity in the ACC and PFC; decreased ability for cognitive processing; decreased activity in left hippocampus; increased activation in left postcentral gyrus and putamen and in the right inferior frontal lobe and middle temporal gyri; decreased activity right middle temporal gyrus, left precuneus, and posterior cingulate gyrus. (After eight weeks of treatment with an antidepressant, certain abnormalities reregulate, and symptoms improve). With improvement, there is reduced cerebral blood flow in the lingual gyrus, left superior temporal gyrus and the right vIFC and also increased blood flow in the left middle occipital gyrus and the inferior parietal cortex. With successful treatment, there is also decreased cerebral blood flow in the ventral dorsal ACC, dorsolateral PFC, and brain stem, and increased cerebral blood flow in the middle cingulate cortex, left hippocampus, parahippocampal gyrus, subcallosal orbital and superior frontal gyri.

The combined results of imaging analysis suggest dysfunction of cortico-striatal-thalamic network: hyperactivity in the RPFC, striatal dysfunction and hippocampus and amygdala activity with left lateralization. It has been suggested hyperactivity in the frontal limbic system and ACC, which process emotional information and anticipate aversive stimuli, result in negative interpretation of social cues.

Individuals with SAD have increases in excitatory glutamatergic activity. The glutamate creatine ratio is 13.2 percent higher than in unaffected individuals. The elevated amygdalae activity is thought to be associated with serotonergic imbalances and disrupted monoaminergic signaling, decreased 5-HT1A receptors, and binding in the amygdalae, ACC, insula, and dorsal raphe nucleus, one or two copies of short SERT alleles, decreased density of the dopamine transporter, decreased binding capacity of the DO receptor, and SSRI-induced desensitization of the postsynaptic D3 receptor.

To induce symptomatic improvement, direct injection of neuropeptides, oxytocin, and vasopressin into the amygdalae of inhabited mice improves and dampens amygdala brain stem communications. Central vasopressin and oxytocin receptors positively influence amygdala activity. One hypothesis is the amygdalae, corticotrophin-releasing factor, and the hypothalamic-pituitary-adrenal axis are hyperactive in SAD.

Sensitization of psychosocial stressors produces greater increases in plasma cortisol. The degree of cortisol elevation correlated with increased social avoidance behavior. Additive genetics accounts for 30 percent of the risk for SAD. The rest is environmental experiences.

Genome-wide linkage with SAD: Chromosome 16 has gene encoding for the norepinephrine transporter. Other genes encoding for SAD include a variant of ABRBI, which encodes for the B-1 adrenergic receptor, two SNPs, and a 3-SNP haplotype in the gene for COMT, a gene encoding for glutamic acid decarboxylase (the rate-limiting enzyme in the synthesis of GABA from glutamate.)

Whoa! All of the above certainly sounds scientific. One can be sure hundreds of researchers in hundreds of laboratories have been toiling away for years hunting down all these molecules, mechanisms, and pathways—the fruits of genuine scientific endeavor.

Many, maybe even most, therapy psychiatrists don't cotton up much to science. Science interferes with their lovely psychodynamic theories and abstractions, the essential framework that justifies their administration of psychodynamic psychotherapy every week for forty-five-minutes for perhaps several years per patient. And neuroscience? Forget it. There is just so much jargon that it's best avoided at all costs since it's so foreign and so complicated.

GLOSSARY

anhedonia. Incapacity to experience interest, enjoyment, or pleasure even in optimal circumstances.

BDNF. A neurotrophic factor sustaining neuron health.

caudate (also called striatum). A paired subcortical structure associated with the basal ganglia. Involved in memory and learning.

CREB (cAMP response element-binding protein). It binds to specific DNA segments, transcribing them to RNA. A transcription factor.

cytokines. Cell signaling molecules that can be associated with injurious inflammatory processes.

dendritic spines. Connecting area on dendrites for axons from other neurons.

dendritic pathology. Decreases in dendritic spine density reducing neural signaling.

dorsolateral prefrontal cortex. Important for working memory and executive functions.

dorsal-medial prefrontal cortex. Important for attention and cognition.

hippocampus. A part of the brain involved in memory formation and storage. Part of the limbic system.

inflammation. The body's response to injury, which can play a role in some chronic diseases.

ion channel. Pore formed of proteins in cell membranes that control passage of ion into and out of neurons.

ketamine. A dissociative anesthetic, which by blocking (antagonizing) the NMDAr, may have therapeutic efficacy for MDD. Also is an abusable drug.

NAC (nucleus accumbens). Part of the basal ganglia playing a central role in reward circuit.

neurogenesis. The process in which new neurons are generated from neural stem cells.

neurotrophic factors. A family of biomolecules, which are peptides or small proteins that support neuron health.

NMDAr (N-methyl-d-aspartate receptor). An ion-channel type for glutamate and glycine.

orbital frontal cortex. A prefrontal cortical region involved in cognitive processing and decision-making.

Parkinson's disease. A neurological disease marked by tremor, muscle rigidity, and slowing of movement.

plasticity. The ability of the brain to modify its own structure and function to adopt to changes in the environment and body.

putamen. Part of the dorsal striatum with caudate nucleus involved in movement.

RNA (ribonucleic acid). Along with DNA, it expresses the gene into proteins required by the cell.

RNA biomarkers. Biomarkers have been used in diagnostic testing for many years. There are subtypes of RNA, mRNA, microRNA, IncRNA that can be measured in the laboratory.

striatum. Critical component of reward system. Is the primary input into the basal ganglia system.

transcription factors. Proteins that bind to specific DNA segments in the nucleus, controlling the copying of DNA into RNA.

ventral striatum. Important for reward system.

CHAPTER 10

Depression

Depression refers to a sadness of mood. Everyone has experienced such a mood at various times, usually as a reaction to unfavorable circumstances or outcomes. So, what's with people diagnosed with depression? Why don't they just get over it like the rest of us? Of course, perhaps the reason they don't or can't is because they're afflicted with character flaws, a penchant for self-indulgence, and self-pity. A passiveness, a lack of initiative, an inclination to avoid responsibility, a total lack of grit and determination. After all, if they can avoid a task or an obligation, it almost always turns out someone else will fill in. Probably the nub of the matter is a flabbiness of will or a lack of willpower? They are always saying stigma should be reduced when referencing mental illness. Did it ever occur to us that they deserve the stigma their lifestyle choices have called forth, the unpleasant emotions they foist on others, the noxious behaviors and symptoms exuding from them? The therapy psychiatrists are right when they entitle their bible *The Diagnostic and Statistical Manual of Mental Disorders.*

Since theirs is the territory for treating mental illness, what is better for these mental problems than psychodynamically oriented psychotherapy? The only way mental patients can be guided, even cajoled to behave like adults, is to undergo a prolonged process of reregulation utilizing weekly (even two to four sessions per week) of psychiatrically administered therapy over several years. Here, the therapy psychiatrist will shine, making incisive, brilliant, probing interpretations that will ultimately revamp the juvenile-like patient who becomes filled with a new wisdom bestowed on them by the therapy psychiatrist.

To the therapy psychiatrist, there is one depression that psychoanalytically oriented psychotherapy cures. If certain patients have different types of depression that do not respond to the therapy psychiatrists' approach, then they are hopeless, they can't be analyzed. They are not worth bothering with!

Actually, what is tragic is that therapy psychiatrists have labeled major depression as *depression,* which causes almost all physicians and the public to confuse it with a minor degree of sad mood, which drives stigma and attendant humiliation that patients must endure in addition to the symptoms of the disease itself.

Anhedonia

What is unique about major depression is its ability to strip the pleasure centers of the brain bare, a metaphorical desert, a joyless wasteland. *Anhedonia* is the loss of the capacity to experience any enjoyment, satisfaction, interest, or humor, the loss of all motivation to fulfill ones wishes, the sense of deadness infiltrating relationships with loved ones. It is a totally involuntary drastic change in mental status. Anhedonia, unlike depression, is not experienced by individuals who don't have the disease. One cannot will oneself into anhedonia. And then what fills the desert? Dread, feelings of doom, terror, and a powerful conviction that there will be no escape. At such a time, suicide takes on a certain logic if no help is forthcoming because it can seem to be the only means of escape.

Depression is the poster child of therapy psychiatrists, an illness impregnated with deep intrapsychic conflicts, according to them. Symptoms are attributed to deep repression of hideous aggressive and sexual impulses that only their own psychoanalytically oriented psychotherapy, characterized by their brilliant interpretations pointed at the deep conflicts and repressions, can alleviate, given persistence of therapy over several years. In some instances, depending on the experience and sensitivity of the psychiatrist, some patients probably benefit. In other instances, it is really hard to ascertain what is going on in therapy. Are there actual results? The patient really is on his or her own.

The cumulative bills for such services will really add up, often necessitating that patients cut spending on other needs. Newer therapies have been scientifically studied—cognitive therapies, behavioral therapies, response-prevention therapies—but they all require special training. It is the extremely rare therapy psychiatrist who bothers with such. It is the lay therapists, MSWs, and PhDs who acquire the expertise. Social workers, like psychiatrists, also provide general psychotherapy, but they do not pompously label it *psychodynamic* or *psychoanalytic*. In most instances, it is the same product the psychiatrists utilize, but at half to a third the cost. (There is no need to cut back on groceries, dining out, hobbies, or necessities for childcare to foot the psychiatrist's therapy bills).

Every ten years, extensive research is conducted to determine the global disability burden caused by 291 separate diseases or injuries. One group of researchers decided to assess the burden of depressive disorders relative to the other 290 diseases or injuries.[21]

As background, they explain:

> Depressive disorders are common mental disorders that occur in people of all ages across would regions. Depression—an overwhelming feeling of sadness and hopelessness that can last for months or years—can make people feel that life is no longer worth living. People affected by depression lose interest in the

21 "Burden of Depressive Disorders by Country, Sex, Age and Year: Findings from the Global Burden of Disease Study 2010," Ferrari, A. J. et al. published Nov. 5, 2013. DOI:10.1371/journal.pmed.1001547).

> activities they used to enjoy and can also be affected by physical symptoms such as disturbed sleep. Major depressive disorder (MDD), also known as clinical depression, is an episodic disorder with a chronic (long-term) outcome and increased risk of death. It involves at least one major depressive episode in which the affected individual experiences a depressed mood almost all day, every day for at least two weeks. Dysthymia is a milder, chronic form of depression that lasts at least two years. People with dysthymia are often described as constantly unhappy. Both these subtypes of depression (and others such as that experienced in bipolar disorder) can be treated with antidepressant drugs and with talking therapies.

In the original study, the researchers quantified the severity of health loss for the 291 diseases and injuries. They statistically devised two specific measurements: years lived with disabilities (YLDs) and disability adjusted life years (DALYs). Depressive disorders were the second-leading cause of YLDs in 2010 (out of the 291 different diseases and injuries). The researchers concluded depressive disorders were a leading cause of disability globally, either directly or through its causation of ischemic heart disease and the complications stemming from the sequelae of suicidal attempts.

They concluded because depression results in such extensive disease burden, it must be treated as a public health priority, and cost-effective interventions needed to be devised to reduce the disease burden. They further amplified the true burden of depressive disorders may be underestimated and also commented there may also be a causal relationship between MDD and strokes, diabetes, and vascular and Alzheimer's disease, although further research is necessary to prove the associations.

By what abnormality of rationality are so-called depressive disorders sliced out of the roster of 291 physical diseases and injuries and labeled mental, which can only detract from the recommended increased emphasis as a public health priority in order to implement cost-effective interventions? We can't escape it. We subconsciously automatically relegate illnesses labeled mental as different from (real) physical illnesses. We have been conditioned to do so for centuries.

In addition to the stigmatization burden, there is also the trivialization burden, both of which mitigate against taking the so-called mental disorders seriously. And don't look toward the psychiatric profession to vigorously seek to discard the whole business of mental terminology. It is a status quo profession. Although it supposedly experts on subconscious and unconscious processes, it is fat and happy with the framework it continues to impose on its patients (*The Diagnostic and Statistical Manual of Mental Disorders*). Change will have to come from patients and their families who are fed up with being slurred.

Scientific Evidence of the Causes of So-Called Depressive Illnesses

Of course, as already mentioned, therapy psychiatrists continue to posit deep psychological conflicts as the cause of depressive illness—just as they have been doing since Freud. In the light of modern neuroscience, it can be said with certainty their so-called psychodynamic theories are really prescientific speculations lacking the proof of rigorous science and are more consistent with dogma or a form of godless religion. It still serves as the theoretical foundation for the practice of many of them. This approach cannot believably be categorized as the practice of medicine, and the medical qualifications of such practitioners are to be seriously questioned.

Brain psychiatrists, over the past two decades, using bona fide actual scientific methods, have been making impressive progress in understanding the physical causes of the disease. Older theories are being supplanted by more comprehensive explanatory ones, largely due to the advances in laboratory techniques and equipment. Initially, it was thought deficiencies in neurotransmitters in the brain were the primary cause, but now it is being learned that the causes arise from the basic working units of the brain itself.

In major depression the very neurons lose adoptability; this is termed a *reduction in plasticity*. Simultaneously the brain is hampered in producing new neurons (neurogenesis), so there is a relative deficiency of them. Neuronal components are reduced in number and function abnormally. There is loss of dendritic spines and connections. There is damage to and loss of synapses. There is reduction in the availability of neurotropic factors (molecules that maintain neuron health and reduction of important subsidiary cells (glial cells) that support and maintain neuron health.

If these dysfunctions persist, neuron cell death spreads (apoptosis). Neurons in the hippocampus and frontal cortex are the most susceptible, the very regions responsible for memory and rational thought. Antidepressant medications, which take several weeks to exert therapeutic efficacy, quite incredibly begin to reverse these destructive changes by promoting neurogenesis and exerting reparative mechanisms to repair neuroplastic degenerations.

Complex pharmacotherapy will be reviewed in a subsequent chapter, but it is important to understand the brain psychiatrist must understand multiple differing specific brain mechanisms and how to employ a number of medications together to readjust specified ones in the directions necessary to promote positive synergistic change. This involves much more than prescribing just one drug and hoping for the best. It involves strategic planning and is a highly specialized endeavor. The current name for this specialist is *clinical psychopharmacologist*.

Ketamine

The physical causes of severe so-called depressive disorders that underlie the impairments in neuroplasticity, reductions in neurogenesis, deficits in synapses, reductions in neurotrophins, and dendritic pathology are complex. Evidence-based neuroscientific research is beginning to outline the basic dysfunctions in brain mechanisms. A major physical dysregulation is neuro-inflammation. The plasma of patients with major depression have excessive levels of cytokines, molecules that upregulate inflammatory processes to the point of injuring tissues for which no such increase would otherwise be called for. Inflammatory markers such as C-reactive protein reach unhealthy levels. With the remission of a severe depressive episode after successful treatment, the levels of cytokines and C-reactive protein normalize.

There is a particular receptor in the brain, the N-methyl-d-aspartate (NMDA) receptor which seems to have particular relevance to major depressive illness. Ketamine, an NMDA antagonist, is currently used in medicine as an anesthetic. If given intravenously in a single dose of 150 mg over a period of one to two hours reverses the entire depressive illness as well as suicidal ideation. (Could it be all those deep unconscious conflicts were magically dissolved by some paranormal experience induced by Ketamine?) Currently ketamine treatment is confined to research protocols, but in the not too distant future, it may bring rapid relief to thousands.

Recent research has demonstrated major depressive illness is associated with anatomical abnormalities in parts of the brain. (Did deep unconscious conflicts sculpt out these abnormalities?) In recent studies, researchers are finding that low hippocampus volume in healthy young girls predicts future major depressive illness. Patients with chronic unremitting depression have an abnormally shaped hippocampus. Additional anatomical abnormalities include reductions in gray matter volume, which harbors the neurons. Another brain area is hypoplastic, the anterior cingulate (Brodmann, 24). This abnormality along with those of the hippocampus, after additional research could serve as biomarkers for major depression on brain scanning, permitting diagnosis from a purely physical image as for strokes, hemorrhages, or tumors.

In summary, Dr. Nasrallah[22] said:

> From healing the mind to repairing the brain, it is well established that depression is associated with loss of dendritic spines and arborizations, loss of synapses, and diminishment of glial cells, especially in the Hippocampus and anterior cingulate. Treating depression, whether pharmacological or somatic, involves reversing these changes by increasing neurotrophic factors, enhancing neurogenesis and gliogenesis, and restoring synaptic and dendritic health and cell survival in the hippocampus and frontal cortex. Treating depression involves brain repair, which is reflected, ultimately, in healing the mind.

Dr. Nasrallah proceeds to discuss the physical treatments for depression. Although pharmacology continues to be a major treatment option, there is a palpable escalation in the use of neuromodulation methods. The oldest of these is electroconvulsive therapy, and even though it has been stigmatized by the media, if given in a center with expertise in its administration, it often saves lives.

A major mechanism through which it ameliorates major depression is through enhancement of hippocampal neurogenesis. In addition, several newer neuromodulation treatments have been developed: transcranial magnetic stimulation, vagus nerve stimulation, transcranial direct-current stimulation, cranial electrotherapy stimulation, and finally DBS (direct brain stimulation).

DBS is of particular interest in that it is a major treatment modality for Parkinson's disease. With slight modifications in placement of the electrode deep into the brain, it is also efficacious for treatment of severe major depression.

---

[22] The author apologizes for losing the specific literature reference for Dr. Nasrallah's commentary.

If the same purely physical treatment that requires the placement of an electrode deep into the brain is used for the physical disorder, Parkinson's disease, then by what gross perversion of reason and logic is depression called mental?

Only the therapy psychiatrists can answer since they originated and continue to use this perverted, stigmatizing, humiliating labeling, slurring the very patients they purport to want to help.

Dr. Eva Redei, PhD, has been developing a blood test to diagnose major depression in the same manner as blood tests used to diagnose diabetes or excessive levels of cholesterol, respectively, a fasting blood sugar or a cholesterol level, both obtained by taking a blood sample, which a certified laboratory then analyzes to assess if the respective levels are elevated.

At a certain agreed-upon elevation of each respectively, a diagnosis of diabetes or hypercholesteremia is made. Dr. Redei and her co-researchers published the scientific study on the new blood test for major depression in *Translational Psychiatry* on September 16, 2014.

In their study, they selected thirty-two patients who had a diagnosis of major depression ascertained by strict criteria from *The Diagnostic and Statistical Manual of Mental Disorders*. The American Psychiatric Association identified another thirty-two subjects who had no symptoms or history of major depression but otherwise were matched to the patients with major depression in terms of other important medical variables: age, medical history, etc.

Before treatment was started—which consisted of a highly specialized form of psychotherapy, cognitive behavioral therapy (CBT)—both the clinically depressed patients and the nondepressed matched individuals (termed control subjects in scientific studies) had blood samples drawn to measure in the laboratory nine different molecules (RNA biomarkers): ADCY3, DGKA, FAM46A, GSF4A/CADM1, KIAA1539, MARCKS, PSME1, RAPH1, and TLR7. After eighteen weeks, in which the clinically depressed individuals received weekly sessions of CBT, blood samples for the RNA biomarkers were again taken from the clinically depressed group and the nondepressed control individuals.

The laboratory result for the nine RNA biomarkers in the clinically depressed group were all different than in the nondepressed controls, clearly distinguishing between the depressed and nondepressed individuals. The results posttreatment with CBT in the patients who had improved with the treatment showed five of the RNA biomarkers had normalized, but three remained abnormal even though the patients had recovered.

The continued abnormal biomarkers are permanently different in people who have major depression in spite of recovery. Why don't people with major depression just snap out of it? All they have to do is change all these abnormal RNA biomarkers back to normal to become just like people who do not have major depression. (Come on now. Concentrate on one biomarker at a time. You can change them if you want to. Just do it—you're not a weakling.)

In a large number of physical illnesses, RNA biomarkers are measured for purposes of expediting diagnosis in the interests of early treatment, which is always preferable to delayed or imprecise diagnosis and untimely treatment.

RNA biomarkers are used to diagnose many cancers, like lung cancer, and cancers of the gastrointestinal track. What form of warped, grossly unscientific logic defines RNA biomarkers in clinical depression as mental—but defines the same class of molecules in other illnesses as physical? If you want an answer, consult the American Psychiatric Association.

Cognitive behavior therapy is termed a *manualized therapy.* It employs specific techniques and programs that are down to earth, and patients can learn, understand, and utilize them to become better. It is the antithesis of vague, rambling psychotherapies many therapy psychiatrists utilize.

This author had a year of postgraduate training to learn CBT. This was beyond the usual three-year psychiatric training program, which is called a residency. Evidence-based CBT has been scientifically proven to help many so-called mental disorders, including major depression.

Most psychiatrists have not had any specialized training in CBT. Most practitioners are doctoral-level psychologists, but unfortunately, there are not enough to go around. Some non-MD therapists claim to be cognitive-behavioral therapists, although they have not had specialized training for it.

Telomeres are strands of protective DNA molecules that cap the tips of all the chromosomes in each cell nucleus. They can be thought of as the plastic caps at the ends of shoelaces (which prevent the laces from unraveling) and similarly prevent the unraveling of the chromosomes.

Telomeres are made up of molecules, termed *base pairs*. As part of the aging process, people generally lose between fourteen and twenty base pairs annually, causing the telomeres to shorten. At a critical juncture, when the telomeres are truncated, the cell will age and die (apoptosis).

The process of shortening of telomeres has been linked to increased risk of some cancers, strokes, vascular dementias, heart disease, obesity, osteoporosis, and diabetes. In a study published online November 12, 2013, in *Molecular Psychiatry*, researchers at Amsterdam's VU University Medical Center conducted a large scientific study on the status of telomeres in major depressive disorders.

There were three groups of individuals who were studied, 1,100 with a current episode of clinical depression, 802 people who had prior episode(s) but were recovered, and 510 who did not have MDD. They drew blood samples from all three groups and submitted them for laboratory analysis of the telomeres. The individuals with MDD current or recovered had eighty-three and eighty-four fewer base pairs in their telomeres than those without the disease.

This is the equivalent of four to six years of excessive aging. Individuals who had chronic severe MDD for two years aged seven to ten years more than the individuals without a history of MDD.

The authors, being just as infected by the treacherous dichotomy as everyone else, call MDD an "emotional stressful condition," a "psychological issue," "psychological distress," and "mental troubles."

> MDD is known to disrupt many physical systems such as hormones; causes suppression of the immune system; changes how nerves work and increases the risk for diseases of aging such as heart disease, Type 2 diabetes, dementia and cancer by having a large detrimental impact on the wear and tear of a person's body resulting in accelerated biological aging.

Other researchers unconnected with the study expressed satisfaction with the quality and size of this study. The study conveys important knowledge that MDD, just like a roster of physical diseases, is associated with accelerated aging via pathological telomere shortening.

Are the shortening telomeres in MDD mental ones, while those in heart disease, diabetes, cancer, and dementia physical ones? Call the American Psychiatric Association to explain the difference.

As the therapy psychiatrists continue to treat their patients afflicted with mental illnesses, mental symptoms, and mental health problems, neurosurgeons in partnership with brain psychiatrists are using new neurosurgical techniques designated *stereotaxic neurosurgery.*

A particular target of this surgery is a brain structure, the nucleus accumbens: a target for deep-brain stimulation in resistant major depressive disorder (*Journal of Molecular Psychiatry*, 2013, 1:17). Cecilia Nauczyciel and her associates investigated the role of the nucleus accumbens in the pathophysiology of MDD. They utilized a specialized form of MRI-diffusion tensor imaging, which takes volume measurements of different brain regions and shows the connections between them.

They enumerated differences in the brains of subjects who have MDD from those who do not (designated *normal).* In a study of forty-eight patients with MDD contrasting seventy-six people without MDD (healthy volunteer subjects), there was a 7 percent reduction in the volume of the frontal lobes in those affected.

A more recent study focused on a brain area, the orbitofrontal area (orbitofrontal cortex). There was a reduction in size of up to 32 percent compared with the controls. In addition, the OFC volumetric abnormalities were associated with less density of neurons and correlated with cognitive disturbances.

Furthermore, there were vascular differences (blood vessels) and a reduction in the density and size of neurons in the dorsolateral prefrontal cortex. An additional finding was the reduction of gray matter (containing the neurons) in the dorsolateral and dorsomedial prefrontal cortex. They point out these findings are linked to functioning abnormalities in depressed subjects. They explain that anhedonia, the loss of the capacity to experience any enjoyment, maintain an interest, or obtain a reward experience from all activities previously important to the patient, as well as the abrupt wall thrown up by the suffering brain to the function of the motivational system are the core of symptoms of MDD. Intensive research has probed for the causes of these abnormalities in the reward and motivational domains of the brain, which the authors describe as being the heart of the suffering experienced by people with MDD.

Why don't people claiming to be depressed just get off their butts? It turns out researchers can produce symptoms similar to those of human depression in rodents. Perhaps the rodents, generally mice, had incompetent mothers causing the formation of deep intrapsychic conflicts in their little mouse ids?

Scientists have subjected certain strains of mice to conditions of chronic stress. They develop depression-like symptoms, including markedly increased passivity, reduction in drive-like activities, including eating and sexual behavior, and retreating from social interactions. Even their body habitus gives off an aura of defeat. They appear to lose the capacity to engage in all reward-seeking behaviors. In other words, they appear to be anhedonic. And, of course, unlike in depressed humans, the brains of the depressed-appearing mice can be directly examined; in the process, the mice are rid of their miserable symptoms (a sort of mouse-style involuntary suicide).

There are a number of physical brain correlates associated with the depressed mice. A deficiency in BDNF (brain-derived neurotrophic factor) in the hippocampus, increased CREB, BDNF, (cAMP response element-binding protein) activity in its role as a transcription factor, and decreased dopamine levels in the NAC (nucleus accumbens), the primary reward circuit in the brain.

If CREB activity in the NAC is disrupted or blocked by a CREB-antagonist, the mice have a marked reduction in anhedonic-like symptoms and resume their normal reward-seeking activities.

Now according to the theories of therapy psychiatry, psychoanalysis would provide a much deeper, permanent cure for these mice, but unfortunately, no mouse has yet graduated from a school of psychoanalysis to administer that therapy to these poor depressed mice.

As in the mouse, the nucleus accumbens and the ventral striatum in which it is situated are the two main actors that allow an individual to experience pleasure and sustain drive and motivation. Of course, there is an overlay of far greater complexity. The NAC receives and sends signals to multiple brain areas involving a plethora of neurotransmitters.

By its functioning normally, it greases the gears, so to speak, which promote well-being by playing roles in regulating appetite, sleep, mood, emotional status, energy, and reward systems.

Clinical studies utilizing DBS (deep-brain stimulation) and PET scans (positron emission tomography) demonstrate a sustained positive effect on NAC functioning in response to successful treatment, including increased metabolism and activation of the caudate, putamen, striatum, and cerebral cortex. These improvements on the scans are inversely related to symptomatology, patients showed renewed drive, motivation, and pleasure sense.

Additional systems also influence motivational capacities. Glutamate is a widely distributed excitatory neurotransmitter that can impact the NAC negatively. Ketamine, an antagonist of the NMDA receptor (N-methyl-D-Aspartate receptor), also influences it.

Administration of ketamine (still an experimental treatment) results in a rapid antidepressant effect in a matter of hours to a few short days, much more rapid than the traditional antidepressants. BDNF (brain-derived neurotrophic factor) is a protein with powerful neurotrophic properties. It plays an important role in efficient brain functioning. This same neurotrophic factor, if deficient in mice, results in behavioral withdrawal, social isolation, and a seeming defeated attitude.

BDNF functions include promoting neuronal growth and differentiation, promoting neuronal survival, facilitating neurotransmission, promoting synaptic formation, function, and plasticity, promoting neurogenesis, and in a feedback loop, increasing its own concentration. BDNF has two receptors: TrkB and neurotropin.

Keeping Neurons Healthy

Brain Derived Neurotrophic Factor (BDNF)

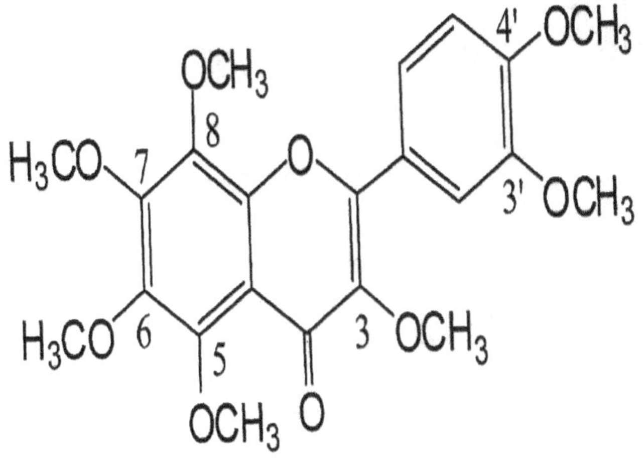

This rather complex molecule is a "nurse" to neurons, plumping them up and keeping their wires and connections (axons, dendrites, synapses) in optimal condition. It also keeps the neuron's self-destruct suicide program on the "off" position.

In summary, the NAC is at the core of the motivational pathways. Poor functioning and the associated structures produce the core symptoms of MDD, anhedonia, and the interruption of motivational drives.

Why don't those people with depression just get off their duffs? All they have to do is reregulate their neurotransmitters, fire up their NACs, and snap out of it. All they have to do is upregulate dopamine, serotonin, and noradrenaline, downregulate glutamate, and manufacture more BDNF. Also, if they really wanted to, they could apply a little lube to the NAC. Come on, don't always take the easy way out—always feeling sorry for yourself. Just push on! Be strong!

Ebola! What does that obvious physical disease have to do with the mental illness of so-called depression? You don't have to call the American Psychiatric Association about this just yet; I doubt if any therapy psychiatrist has the slightest idea.

Researchers at the US Army Medical Research Institute of Infectious Diseases the University of Virginia and Horizon Discovery Inc. reasoned, rather than inventing new compounds to treat Ebola, it would be much less expensive to try already approved drugs against the virus. A benefit is the side effects of the drugs are already a known quantity. They began their research with 2,635 different medications. Each was individually tested on a version of the Ebola virus that was engineered to turn green when exposed to ultraviolet light.

A drug was considered worth further researching if it reduced the green signal by 40 percent and did not harm a sample of normal cells derived from the kidneys of African green monkeys. A total of 171 compounds made the first cut. From them, the researchers selected the thirty most promising and tested them further in kidney cells and human liver cancer cells.

They determined twenty-five drugs were able to block the entry of the virus into cells by more than 90 percent. After further elimination trials, they ended up with two compounds that were the most beneficial. The first compound allowed seven of ten mice to survive a full month; for the second, ten out of ten survived. For comparison, all the mice in the control groups died within nine days.

Further testing will be required on nonhuman primates before the drugs can receive an FDA indication for the treatment of patients infected with Ebola, but it is hoped that repurposing these two approved drugs will reduce risk, time, and cost.

The two compounds out of the original 2,635 are a blood pressure medication not available in the United States, Vascor, and the commonly used antidepressant Zoloft (sertraline).

Why is a drug that is efficacious against the Ebola virus, when it is used to treat MDD, labeled a mental drug treating so-called mental illness? Don't bother to ask the therapy psychiatrists. They are invested in maintaining the antiquated, unscientific, stigmatizing, humiliating, slurring frame of reference as indicated in the title of their bible: *The Diagnostic and Statistical Manual of Mental Disorders.*

Another topic worthy of review is the relationship of so-called mental illnesses to the physical diseases of the brain: strokes, Parkinson's disease, and cognitive and memory decline. Minimal cognitive impairment (MCI) is a less severe form of cognitive impairment that greatly increases the risk for Alzheimer's disease.

Swedish researchers[23] compared 140,688 people with depression to 421,943 controls over a period extending up to twenty-five years.

During that period, 3,260 cases of Parkinson's disease occurred. The incidence of Parkinson's disease was tripled for the group who had MDD. The lead author, Professor Peter Nordstrom, a professor of geriatrics at Umea University in Sweden, hypothesized depression damages the brain, causing the increase in Parkinson's disease. He clarified the overall risk of developing Parkinson's is relatively small. Another researcher explained the link that affects the neurotransmitters; dopamine and serotonin may play an important role.

There are eight known risk factors for Alzheimer's disease. Seven of the risks are older age, female gender, genetic predisposition, lipoprotein A, cardiovascular disease, Down syndrome, and head injury. The eighth is MDD, which doubles the risk.

In a study[24] conducted at Albert Einstein School of Medicine, 528 subjects free of MCI underwent annual neurological examinations, neuropsychological testing, standardized assessments of activities of daily living, and depression screening for a period of years.

Of these, seventy-three later developed MCI. They were found to have had the highest levels of perceived stress, which is correlated with MDD. In a second study, 706 participants were followed over

---

[23] *The New York Times*, May 20, 2015)

[24] *Neurology Reviews*, 2013, 21 (10.8).

time to evaluate the influence of pain, levels of stress, and depression on cognitive function.

After adjusting statistically for all the variables, depression was most correlated with cognitive decline, including MCI and Alzheimer's disease. A study appearing in the *Journal of the American Heart Association*, "Changes in Depressive Symptoms and Incidences of First Stroke Among Middle-Aged and Older U.S. Adults,"[25] had the objective to further elucidate the previously demonstrated finding that depressive symptoms predict an increase in the incidence of strokes and cerebral vascular accidents (CVA).

A nationally representative cohort of American adults older than fifty years of age with no prior history of stroke, 16,178 individuals, were followed for ten years (2000–2010) with regular medical and psychiatric examinations to determine symptom levels.

During that period, 1,192 strokes occurred. Participants with high levels of major depression had 2.71 strokes (utilizing systematic statistical methods) for every one stroke occurring in the control participants without MDD.

Successful treatment of the MDD did reduce the stroke incidence, although not completely to the level of the control (healthy) participants. The authors explained the increased incidence of stroke in those with MDD is caused by the accumulation of vascular damage, increased inflammatory processes, and possibly other biological abnormalities in those with MDD. They ended their article with a plea:

> This study, in conjunction with other work confirming that depressive symptoms are causally related to stroke risk, suggests that clinicians should seek to identify and treat depressive symptoms as early as possible relative to their onset, before adverse consequences begin to accumulate.

---

[25] 5/13/2015 doi: 10.1161/JAHA.115: 001923.

However, these well-intentioned researchers may be whistling Dixie. For as long as so-called depression is characterized as a so-called mental illness, it will continue to be taken less seriously than the real, physical illnesses. Thanks to the pervasive influence of the therapy psychiatrists, most physicians still don't believe depression is a real (physical) illness, often neglecting to evaluate for it, let alone treat it effectively.

Two specialties focus on diseases of the brain: neurology and psychiatry. Neurology is a true medical specialty. It researches and studies the physical dimensions of the brain scientifically to learn as much as possible to facilitate effective diagnosis of a spectrum of neurological diseases such as epilepsy, cerebral vascular accidents, multiple sclerosis, myasthenia gravis, and a roster of additional neurological diseases. In its attitude toward the practice of neurology, it adheres firmly to the medical model, linking symptoms and diseases to real, observable, tangible physical abnormalities underlying symptoms and diseases.

Neurologists are all brain neurologists, that is, full-fledged physicians, which are found in all medical specialties from allergy to specialists treating Zollinger-Ellison syndrome.

There is only one really odd-duck specialty: therapy psychiatry. Most of its practitioners really didn't want to go to medical school or take clinical courses in medicine, neurology, pediatrics, and obstetrics-gynecology, but all were mandatory in medical school.

But since Freud was a physician, medical school is de rigueur, a distasteful rite of passage. As soon as possible, they all dispense with the concerted study of medicine and its rather complex requirements, conducting a competent physical examination, knowing the symptoms of multiple diseases, making a scientifically informed diagnosis and differential diagnosis, and acquiring an in depth, up-to-date knowledge of the plethora of laboratory tests—and how to order and then interpret them.

Instead, their vision is of a higher nature, sophisticated philosophy, and deep psychoanalytic psychotherapy. They will remold those wretched individuals, their patients, by means of expertly applied psychodynamic techniques, creating a new human, who is elevated in wishes and desires and free of the baser instincts and drives!

It was up to a distinguished neurologist, Andres Kanner, MD, professor of clinical neurology at the University of Miami's Miller School of Medicine, to elucidate the relationship between mental problems and physical illnesses.

Of course, the treacherous dichotomy perpetuated by therapy psychiatrists causes nearly everybody, including physicians, to consciously and certainly unconsciously classify mental illnesses as a distinct class of problems, widely separated from the real physical diseases.

A corollary of this psychiatric construct is that real physical illnesses aren't affected by mental problems. How can such mental problems affect real physical illnesses in which physical dysfunctions cause symptoms?

Does an ethereal breeze cause damage to the rock of Gibraltar? Yes, it took a brain neurologist to acknowledge that neurological illnesses and so-called mental illnesses have a bidirectional physical interaction, making it clear this does not involve the ether on the part of mental disorders, but the dysregulation of the physical brain operating in both directions.

There are not two separate compartments. There is only one, and it is called the brain! The brain is a physical organ!

No sane physician would claim seizure disorders (epilepsy) are not physical illnesses. Although there are many subtypes, the most well-known type is the generalized tonic clonic seizure. The individual loses consciousness, and the muscles contract throughout the body. Contraction of the jaw muscles causes biting of the tongue. The patient falls to the ground. After ten or twenty seconds, the tonic (contraction) phase transitions to the tonic-clonic phase in which the limbs jerk back and forth. Patients gradually regain consciousness after minutes to hours, termed the post-ictal phase, during which they are confused and disoriented. The most important recent progress in epilepsy research has been the identification of genetic abnormalities, particularly those which cause abnormal ion-channel function, influencing neuronal homeostasis.

A real puzzlement is how can MDD, characterized by the American Psychiatric Association as a mental disorder, have any relationship to or impact on grand mal epilepsy? Can a wisp of a mental thought or emotion, which can be controlled by keeping up your mental health, possibly bear any relationship to an individual who is unconscious and violently shaking on the ground?

Dr. Kanner reviews the facts of the underlying *physical* basis for MDD. He comments on the genetic predisposition of psychiatric disorders. For example, first-degree relatives of subjects with epilepsy have a two to three times greater risk compared to the general population for also developing MDD.

The lifetime risk rises to eight to nine times higher for bipolar disorder. The heritability estimate for MDD is 33–42 percent and 68–80 percent for bipolar disorder. This heritability is explained on the basis of multiple genes with variable penetrance. And this genetic modeling is the same for many common physical illnesses, cardiovascular disease, some cancers, etc.

He reviews neurobiological pathogenic mechanisms operant in psychiatric disorders, which yield such hyperexcitability. These include an increase in glutamatergic and a decrease in GABA-ergic neurotransmission in the brain; a decrease in serotonergic activity, which has been shown to facilitate seizure occurrence in animal models of epilepsy; a hyperactive hypothalamic-pituitary-adrenal axis, which is associated with decreased serotonergic and increased glutamatergic activity and structural changes in the brain, including bilateral hippocampal atrophy and atrophy of various frontal lobe structures, and inflammatory disturbances in the brain, which through glutamatergic mechanisms have also been identified as pathogenic mechanisms of seizures.

Dr. Kanner observes it is the commonality of so many pathogenic mechanisms that are responsible for the high comorbid occurrence of these disorders. That is why individuals with MDD have a significantly greater incidence of epilepsy than individuals free of MDD.

GLOSSARY

dorsal system of brain. An alternative system to the right brain-left brain dichotomy, which divides the brain into dorsal (top) and ventral (bottom) systems. If the ventral system is upregulated, the dorsal system has decreased activity.

estradiol. The primary female sex hormone important in the regulation of the estrous and menstrual female reproductive cycles. It is essential for the development and maintenance of female reproductive tissues.

estradiol high phase. Greater concentrations are available.

estradiol low phase. Lesser concentrations associated with the premenstrual phase of the menstrual cycle, the postpartum period, and menopause transition (perimenopause).

hippocampus. During estradiol low phase, its function is suppressed which may impair learning.

hyperactive state. Overactivity of a given bodily process.

limbic system. During estradiol low phase, there is decreased modulation by the cortex, resulting in increased emotionality.

susceptibility. During estradiol low phase, there is greater vulnerability to psychosocial stress and the occurrence of MDD (major depressive disorder).

ventral system of brain. Inclined to be hyperactive in some instances during estradiol law phase. Components include amygdala, insula, ventral striatum, and ventral regions of cingulate gyrus and prefrontal cortex.

CHAPTER 11

Depression, Epilepsy, and Pregnancy

As a rule, over the past several decades, most neurologists do not attempt to detect psychiatric comorbidities in epilepsy treatment. (This is not a surprise since the mental health characterization of these illnesses by psychiatry does not lend itself to other physicians taking psychiatric symptoms or illnesses seriously.) To most real physicians, mental health sounds something like dental health, which can be maintained by flossing regularly.

Gradually, however, at least on the part of some enlightened neurologists, there has been recognition of the interplay of pathogenic mechanisms that are responsible for the very high comorbidity between epilepsy and psychiatric disorders, particularly mood disorders like MDD. For patients who develop epilepsy, there is a much greater load of psychiatric illness before its onset than in the general population.

Epileptics have a sevenfold higher risk of developing schizophrenia. Children with ADHD have a nearly fourfold higher risk of developing epilepsy. Similarly, for most major psychiatric disorders, there is an increased risk of developing epilepsy.

In turn, individuals who develop epilepsy have a three times higher risk of developing psychiatric disorders subsequently. A particular concern is the development of serious suicidality after the onset of epilepsy, which can lead to fatality (*post-ictal suicidal ideation.*)

A prior history of a severe mood illness requiring hospitalization is a marker for serious suicidal risk after the onset of epilepsy, particularly in the twenty-four hours after a seizure occurs. (This is an emergency situation.)

Given the high lifetime prevalence of psychiatric illness in those who are diagnosed with epilepsy, nearly 40 percent compared to 10 percent in the general population, a few enlightened neurologists make an effort to screen for psychiatric symptoms utilizing specifically designed scales containing relevant psychiatric symptoms for the patient to respond to.

One of these is the Neurologic Disorders Depression Inventory in Epilepsy (NDDI-E) for MDD and the patient's health questionnaire. After utilizing these screening instruments, a more in-depth evaluation is always recommended to make a psychiatric diagnosis and establish the duration and existence of psychiatric comorbidities by taking a life-time psychiatric history and inquiring about the presence of psychiatric illness in first-degree relatives.

It is felt to be essential at the time of the initial evaluation of the seizure to identify those who will be at risk for future psychiatric illness, including their most serious complication: completed suicide. Such a methodical approach on the part of neurologists in practice rarely occurs. Psychiatrists are mostly of the therapy type and are incapable of having meaningful communications about the psychiatric-neurological nexus.

Epileptics and their families also must be made aware of the increased risk of an occurrence of a psychiatric disorder, and they must be encouraged to report it to the treating physician.

Antiepileptic medications (anticonvulsants) are utilized for both seizure disorders and bipolar mood disorders. There is overlap of some anticonvulsants, which are helpful for both disorders. Others may have an advantage for mood disorders.

A high level of expertise is required for individual treatments. Often two anticonvulsants in various combinations may need to be worked out for a given patient.

There are multiple choices. On the whole, certain anticonvulsants may be less optimal for mood disorders: barbiturates, topiramate, levetiracetam benzodiazepines, vigabatrin, and Zonisamide—and valproic acid, carbamazepine, oxcarbazepine, and lamotrigine. Pregabalin and gabapentin are better for anxiety symptoms.

Discontinuation of an anticonvulsant that is stabilizing a mood or anxiety disorder can lead to a breakout of a psychiatric episode, including suicidality. It is in the prescription of anticonvulsants that a high degree of collaboration is essential between a neurologist and a psychiatrist.

Unfortunately, if the neurologist collaborates with a therapy psychiatrist, major errors in the use of these medications becomes a high likelihood, and an eruption of symptoms, untoward side effects, and disruptions in daily routines is likely.

It is not clear if neurologists know the distinction between a therapy versus a brain psychiatrist and that they should only collaborate with a brain psychiatrist to ensure their patients receive appropriate psychiatric diagnosis and safe, sophisticated psychopharmacology in conjunction with ongoing neurological treatment.

In the utilization of anticonvulsant medications, there is always puzzlement. Why are these obviously physical medications, which treat physical neurological illnesses, suddenly becoming mental treatments when used to treat so-called mental illnesses. This is another question the American Psychiatric Association ought to answer.

Pregnancy, Major Depression, and Antidepressants

Andrew Solomon is a professor of psychology at Columbia University. He is the author of *The Noonday Demon: An Atlas of Depression*. He recently wrote an update to the final chapter of the book, a version of which, *The Secret Sadness of Pregnancy with Depression*, appeared in the *New York Times Sunday Magazine* on May 28, 2015.

Professor Solomon has MDD, and his book tells the story of his personal experience with the illness. When he became a father, he was fearful of being somehow inadequate for fatherhood and that he would lose his own stability going through such a momentous change. He worried he would pass on a genetic legacy of depression.

In reality, having children transformed his depression. It gave him new priorities, new concerns, new goals, and in some ways, a new sense of peace.

His interest was tweaked. For his doctoral research, he interviewed twenty-four women over a period of five years about their experiences of motherhood with particular emphasis on the changes parents undergo. Many of his subjects had experienced depression in the context of their pregnancies and new status as mothers.

He ventured into the emergent field of reproductive psychiatry, reading dozens of studies and talking to experts. He comments on postpartum depression in the past two decades have received some recognition, but antenatal depression (depression suffered during pregnancy), which affects 10–15 percent of expectant women, is still largely ignored by obstetricians. Some of these women have had undiagnosed depression for years without adequate diagnosis or treatment. Others discontinue antidepressants upon learning they are pregnant, often at the urging of the obstetrician.

This brings up the first talking point. The pregnant woman and her obstetrician may believe continuing a medication, which they both believe will be potentially harmful to the fetus, for merely a mental illness is medically inadvisable. Also militating against treatment of depression during the post-pregnancy period is the pervasive stigma of being depressed when they should be expectantly looking forward to motherhood with a host of positive attitudes and fantasies. Professor Solomon notes women who have antenatal depression can even be characterized as heartless as they struggle with the illness that casts a shadow over all the positive aspects of the pregnancy for them.

His article described the approach toward depression and its treatment with antidepressants on the part of an assistant professor at an eastern medical school. The physician who specializes in high-risk pregnancy has campaigned to expose the dangers of antidepressants for pregnant women.

On his website, Common Health, he writes:

> Imagine for a moment that a virus started affecting 5 percent of all pregnant women—200,000 US pregnancies per year. Imagine that it caused significant pregnancy complications. More than 10 percent of those infected with the virus would miscarry; up to 20 percent or more would have preterm birth, and 30 percent of newborns would show the effect of the exposure in days after birth. It would be considered a public health emergency. Yet this epidemic is happening … it is the epidemic of antidepressant drug exposure during pregnancy.

When Professor Solomon spoke to this obstetrician, he compared the SSRIs (selective serotonin reuptake inhibitors like Prozac, Zoloft, and Lexapro) to thalidomide and how they were used due to the undue influence of the pharmaceutical industry.

It is clear this obstetrician does not believe that there is a disease of depression, which can greatly complicate the course of pregnancy and require medical treatment. To him, so-called mental illness is evidently a myth, and by urging all pregnant women to go off antidepressants, there can be no doubt he is promoting suffering, injury, and misery on the part of women who must be on antidepressants.

Although this physician is violently violating his Hippocratic oath, this author cannot blame him. The fault lies in the jurisdiction of the American Psychiatric Association, which perpetuates the treacherous mental-physical dichotomy.

The greatest tragedy is therapy psychiatry, which does not forcefully educate there are subtypes of depression and degrees of severity—and certainly for the more severe forms of depression, the brain is highly physically dysregulated. Instead, they sit in their lounge chairs doing deep psychoanalytic psychotherapy.

Solomon goes on to shed a rational light on the issue of antidepressant use in pregnancy. He notes the SSRIs are one of the most studied class of drugs in pregnancy. They have acknowledged side effects: heightening the risk of miscarriage, preterm birth, and low birth weight. Up to 30 percent of babies exposed in utero to an SSRI develop a condition called neonatal adoption syndrome with symptoms of poor sucking response and respiratory distress, although the symptoms are transitory. The Food and Drug Administration issued a black-box warning for SSRIS, the strongest possible warning for a medication, in 2006, but it was withdrawn in 2011. He describes new research looking into the possible longer-term harmful effects of SSRIs.

One researcher, Dr. Jay Gingrich at Columbia-Presbyterian School of Medicine, has commented that the immediate postpartum effects the high-risk pregnancy obstetrician was so focused on are usually insignificant, but there are open research issues about hypothetical impacts on the developing brain during fetal development, early childhood, and even adolescence. Research is being undertaken to elucidate both positive and negative effects of antidepressants.

There is the conundrum in which negative outcomes are caused by medication or the depressive illness itself. Professor Solomon warns, recalling the Hippocratic oath, that doctors who encourage depressed pregnant women to white-knuckle it can cause grave harm by stopping a prescription for antidepressants or not writing one.

One tragic case was reviewed at the beginning of his article. An accomplished teacher married at thirty-seven and became pregnant. She had struggled with depression on a chronic basis. Medications and psychotherapy did offer her some relief. As soon as she learned she was pregnant, having read of a possible danger to the fetus, she discontinued the antidepressant, but she did continue to see the psychiatric nurse practitioner who had prescribed it. As time passed, she became more and more preoccupied that the fetus had a major defect. She was unable to gain reassurance from genetic testing and multiple ultrasounds that showed the fetus was apparently developing normally. She became more and more obsessed, spending hours online scrutinizing for details of what can go wrong for a fetus. Her sleep deteriorated, and she started having severe nocturnal attacks of sheer panic, becoming completely convinced her baby was fatally flawed. Finally, she left a voice mail to her mother that she couldn't make it. She jumped to her death from the sixteenth floor of a building when she was six and a half months pregnant. Her mother, in thinking of this grievous tragedy, was left with the pain of a choice not taken: if her daughter had only stayed on her medication or at least gotten back on it sooner!

Professor Solomon evidently felt it was important to give a balanced view of the pros and cons of not treating or treating utilizing antidepressant medications. Untreated depression and anxiety during pregnancy have been linked in multiple studies to miscarriage, preeclampsia, preterm birth, neonatal complications, and smaller newborns. The depressive episode itself can be complicated by an increase in obsessive symptoms and surges in the stress hormone cortisol. Cortisol crosses the placental barrier and reaches the fetus. The uterine artery that feeds the placenta may have diminished blood flow. He quotes a study in which the children of mothers who were highly anxious when they were nineteen weeks pregnant showed reduced gray matter in the cerebral cortex (the brain matter that contains the neurons) at ages six through nine. Additional studies found untreated anxiety during pregnancy is correlated with higher levels of anxiety symptoms at four years of age and raised cortisol levels in adolescence. Other scientists have reported depression during pregnancy can alter the newborn's amygdala, a brain region that regulates emotion, memory, and decision-making. Data also indicate high stress levels during pregnancy are associated with cognitive impairment and slowed language development.

The greatest fear of clinically depressed women during pregnancy is they might hurt their infant after birth. The vast majority—even if untreated—do not, but the symptoms of depression result in impaired capacity to bond with, relate to, and attend to the details of the care required. This results in torturous guilt.

Professor Solomon concluded his article with information

he obtained from Elizabeth Fitelson, MD, a prenatal specialist at Columbia-Presbyterian School of Medicine. During an extensive interview, she stresses the importance of taking a systemic view. She pays attention to the mom's capacity not just to bear a child but to care for it. She assesses what's worse for the baby—the mom's depression or the medication to treat it—and bears in mind the mom's symptom level and suffering. Considerations include past history of depression, depression severity, a history of comorbid disorders like substance abuse or eating disorders, and symptomatic response when stopping medication in the past. She has had patients who went off their medication, experienced catastrophic depression, were unable to cope, and terminated their pregnancies. At the opposite pole, she has had patients who remained on medication, had a child with deficiencies, and blamed that decision, experiencing a penumbra of regret and guilt. Statistically for the women she sees in consultation, 10 percent don't need medication, 20 percent require it, and for 70 percent, it's a venture into the unknowable.

The case of Margaret is reported in detail. She worked in the financial-services industry in Manhattan, and she had a significant history of clinical depression in her family. Her grandmother committed suicide before she was born, and her mother, who she vividly remembers sitting in her chair and crying, jumped in front of a subway train when she was ten. She was at the scene of the September 11, 2001, attack on the World Trade Center, and though not injured herself, she began having panic attacks, subsequently relieved by an SSRI, Paxil.

When she became pregnant, she decided she should stop it. Symptoms returned: loss of interest in things, irritability, crying, not wanting to get out of bed, and complete loss of energy or desire to do anything. When her daughter was born, she continued to be short-tempered and disengaged. She realized she was not bonding with her infant and also might be alienating her husband. When her daughter was three months old, she made the decision to go back on antidepressants, a combination therapy of Zoloft and Wellbutrin, and was relieved she could then begin to bond with her daughter. This first pregnancy and its aftermath she experienced were so traumatic that she waited ten years before considering a second pregnancy. This time, there was no thought of going off antidepressants. Her obstetrician was skeptical of her decision, an attitude, she has learned, that is prevalent among obstetricians regarding remaining on or starting antidepressants. She was not swayed by the obstetrician.

Her second pregnancy went beautifully, and she enjoyed every moment. After the birth of her second daughter, it was instant bonding. Margaret, for a period, felt guilty about remaining on the antidepressants during pregnancy, but she transitioned ultimately to feeling guilty she had remained off her medication during the first pregnancy.

Realizing the cost of MDD in her family tree, she had been fearful she might follow the suicidal trajectory of both her grandmother and mother. To her enormous relief, due to the feeling of control over her illness the medication had given her, for the first time, she felt optimistic she would not attempt suicide in the future, and neither would her daughters. "I'm just so happy that I know it's not going to kill me the way I used to assume it could, and it's not going to kill my daughters either."

Professor Solomon concludes:

> I was deeply moved by my conversations with the women whose experiences I drew on in this article, most of whom felt that their struggles had not been validated. They thought their despondent pregnancies were bizarre, outlying experiences. Some had been too ashamed to tell their husbands, their doctors, their mothers—and many of them spoke to me with evident pain when recalling what they had been through. To celebrate an experience that started in secret pain is no easy task, and mothers who had antenatal depression described how it cast a pall over motherhood.

Professor Solomon's thoughtful article illustrates how MDD can disastrously impact two individuals simultaneously. By continuing to refer to MDD disorder as a mental health problem, the facilitation of the trivialization, minimization, and stigmatization of the mother's suffering by most physicians, including obstetricians, is assured. One must implore the American Psychiatric Association to consider how this classification promotes waves of suffering in pregnant women across the entire nation. That organization must take stock. Their classification of future mother's with MDD as mentally ill must finally and rapidly be reappraised.

Women in general have a higher incidence of MDD than males, and therefore, they bear the stigmatization and humiliation of being labeled mentally ill in a greater degree. Increased vulnerability for MDD begins in puberty and only declines at the end of perimenopause. The leading hypothesis for women's increased susceptibility to MDD are the influence of female gonadal steroids, especially a major circulating estrogen, estradiol. It interacts with neurotransmitter and mood-regulatory systems as well life stress by influencing emotional processing and the encoding and retrieving of emotional information. Cortisol, the chief stress hormone, which is regulated by the hypothalamic-pituitary-adrenal axis, is influenced by it. Ultimately neurotransmission and neuro circuits are similarly influenced.

The periods of greatest vulnerability for emotional dysregulation are the premenstrual phase of the menstrual cycle, postpartum periods, and menopause transition (perimenopause).[26] Greater activity in the ventral system of the brain, including the amygdalae, insula, ventral striatum, and ventral regions of the cingulate gyrus and prefrontal cortex are particularly important for the identification of the emotional significance of a stimulus and production of an emotional response to it. Psychosocial stress is associated with heightened activity in these ventral systems paired with decreased activity in the dorsal system. A hyperactive state of the ventral system is associated with increased susceptibility to depressive symptoms and

[26] These are the times when estradiol levels are at their lowest.

MDD. Functional neuroimaging studies in premenstrual women have demonstrated significant differences in cortical activation for negative emotional stimuli during high versus low estradiol phases, suggesting estradiol modulates limbic activity from the top down. Studies of postmenopausal women show decreases in amygdalae activation relative to younger women, which is consistent with the effect of high estradiol levels on the emotional regulatory circuits.

Psychosocial stress combined with lower levels of estradiol may impair learning by suppressing the hippocampus in addition to increasing vulnerability to mood dysregulation by its influence on amygdalae responsiveness. In summary, changing levels of estradiol across the menstrual cycle, postpartum period, and perimenopause have a significant impact on emotional reactivity, cognitive mechanisms, and vulnerability to clinical depression. The American Psychiatric Association owes it to half our population to decide if these women are mentally ill because of symptoms springing from their hormonal cycles. Do they have mental health problems? Should they continue to be stigmatized and humiliated because of a purely physical process, the fluctuation of an important hormone, estradiol, which results in symptomatology and suffering? Is estradiol a mental phenomenon?

CHAPTER 12

Depression, the Elderly, and the Young

The golden years are not so golden for those who develop or have had MDD in this last phase of life. Unfortunately, the medical community on the whole is very insensitive to the symptoms of depression, largely ignoring its presence while focusing on the physical symptoms and illnesses of their patients. After all, a mental symptom or illness does not seem important enough when you are treating the *real* physical symptoms and diseases of patients, which obviously are so detrimental to their quality of life.[27]

It is a significant undertaking to diagnose and treat MDD in the elderly, requiring effort, specialized knowledge, and an extended commitment. Many elderly people dwell in the shadows, withdrawn, socially isolated, devoid of pleasurable experiences, and even suicidal.

Only brain psychiatrists are medically competent enough to properly diagnose and treat the elderly depressed, particularly if they specialize in geriatric psychiatry.

Legions of elderly people, who generally suffer in silence, have unrecognized symptoms that erode the quality of their lives. But who notices a withdrawn, quiet old person? It's just part of old age! The symptoms of major depression are no more benign than in younger

[27] And even the 20 percent of the time a primary care physician recognizes clinical depression, he or she may not know who to refer to. An MSW? A psychologist? A therapy psychiatrist?

people, and due to their age, their last memory of life may be of the agonizing depressed state: feeling isolated and alone even when with others, subsisting in a gray-colorless zone of anhedonia, inexplicably unable to enjoy any activity or interest, feeling trapped and hopeless, unable to envision their miserable lives will ever attenuate (and many will die in this mode), feeling exhausted all the time, being enveloped by guilt because they cannot function as they know they should, feeling like a hideous burden to their families, and often hoping, even though most but not all[28] are disinclined to attempt suicide, that they would just die!

Because they often have periods of unexplained irritability and anxiety, they may fear they will antagonize or alienate those on whom they are even more dependent emotionally. And all this largely unspoken since clinical depression impairs and closes off communication. It is essentially a brain lock into a new mental universe of horrors and fears, in which all prior positive aspects of life are locked out!

For that rare breed of primary care physician who is cognizant there is a real illness called MDD, the first responsibility is to use a screening instrument, a validated scale like the Patient Health Questionnaire 9 that reflects diagnostic criteria. It is critical to identify warning signs supporting urgent intervention including severe or worsening symptoms, suicidality, and impairment in daily functioning.

Screening must be followed by a competent full evaluation. For this, the brain psychiatrist is best equipped due to his specialized expertise in neuroscience, diagnosis, differential diagnosis, and neurology. A long list of medical and neurological diseases must be considered. Are there specific coexisting medical and neurological illnesses? Abnormal laboratory studies? All the patient's medications must be evaluated. Are there questions of drug interactions? Cognitive functions must be assessed, which if significantly impaired, may indicate accelerated brain aging, which perpetuates depression and

---

[28] Elderly white males are at high risk for suicide.

raises the risk of dementia. Metabolic conditions such as thyroid abnormalities, electrolyte imbalance, and vitamin deficiencies are critical considerations.

First-line treatment for the elderly include skilled, cautiously prescribed medications (geriatric pharmacology) and practical psychotherapy, which emphasizes coping skills, helping the patient understand the illness as a brain dysregulation rather than a weakness, and a cause deserving pernicious guilty feelings.

The psychopharmacology of elderly people requires a sophisticated, delicate touch and a deep knowledge of drug interactions because they may be on a large number of medications for various illnesses. An important objective is to start with generally lower doses and increase the dosage with an eye toward minimizing side effects.

As is the case for younger people, sometimes combinations of medications for MDD may be necessary, and employing them requires specialized skills.

The Young

MDD cares not a whit about the ages of the individuals in which it occurs. At the other end of the age spectrum are the very young: toddlers, children, adolescents, and young adults.

Researchers have found worrying amounts of psychotropic drug use in younger and younger patients.[29] Employing information from the Medicaid Analytic Extract from thirty-six states, they determined a growing number of preschool children are being prescribed psychotropic medications. The researchers find the numbers particularly alarming because they indicate that doctors are increasingly willing to prescribe psychotropic drugs to young patients who might benefit from behavior therapy. The article explains how it is possible that some of these children may have brain injuries or insults such as traumatic brain injuries, fetal alcohol syndrome, or other conditions for which treatment is not being provided.

---

[29] "Bell Ringer," posted April 14, 2015, by Sam Rolley.

> If the medications are being solely used for behavioral control, then it seems clear that we need to better assess children to see if they might be better served by the use of evidence-based behavioral interventions.

One can easily infer that psychotropic drug use is not justified in children, and it may interfere with real treatments for actual physical diseases. If a child has some behavioral disturbance, the treatment should be psychotherapy.

This author cannot criticize the researchers or authors quoted in the article. They are unfortunately ignorant of the real physical basis for the so-called mental illnesses. The painful fact is the psychiatric profession grooves by keeping these illnesses in the stigmatizing mental category because this serves as the rationale for doing long-term weekly forty-five-minute therapy sessions, even with youngsters. It is only human to favor that which provides your income even if you are stigmatizing and humiliating your patients by labeling them as mental cases. Even toddlers are so labeled!

If you are able to appreciate the evidence with an open mind, you will understand the physical causality of the major so-called mental illnesses. It would be grossly inappropriate and negligent to deny psychotropic medication to a youngster if there is a medical rationale to prescribe it. The issue is who will decide? In neurology, there are seizure disorders that occur in infancy and early childhood. Let's transpose the statement about alarm regarding psychotropic drug use into one about use of neurological drugs. There is a large overlap of drugs used for psychiatric and neurological illnesses, the same medications in many instances.

Neurologists prescribe a host of medications for infants and young children, such as valproic acid, lamotrigine, ethosuximide, topiramate, levetiracetam, and others. Valproic acid, topiramate, and lamotrigine are also commonly prescribed for specific so-called mental disorders. Are they real medicines when a neurologist prescribes them—but not if a child with a so-called mental illness could benefit? Does the mental patient go without medical treatment across the board—though they will be permitted to react or talk in psychotherapy?

The critical issue when prescribing for infants and young children is that the prescriber is a competent clinician with a depth of training and experience who does a thorough evaluation before prescribing. The provider should be a pediatric neurologist or child and adolescent brain psychiatrist. Unfortunately, psychiatry lags behind neurology in the relative rigorousness of their approaches. Nearly every neurologist will order laboratory tests and an electroencephalogram and keep up with the most up-to-date pharmacological treatments. There is less certainty about psychiatrists. Are they conducting a thorough diagnostic interview? Are they using the psychiatric equivalent of an EEG to facilitate diagnosis? The Mini-International Neuropsychiatric Interview greatly facilitates the diagnostic process, and there is a child version. Are they emphasizing evidence-based pharmacological treatments to provide optimal pharmacological treatment for their young patients?

In the absence of clinical competence and experience in the evaluation of young patients—and rusty or absent medical and pharmacological skills—there is a wide latitude for mistaken diagnosis and scattershot, inappropriate prescribing. That is the crux of the matter, which is a far different emphasis than proclaiming so-called psychotropic medications should not be prescribed to youngsters. The problem is in the practitioners and not in the medications. Unfortunately, there is a far greater variation in competence among psychiatrists than neurologists that traces back to the split identity of psychiatry. Are they therapists? Are they physicians? It's only the rare gifted practitioner who can maintain high levels of competence in such divergent methods of treatment simultaneously over time.

"Mental-Health Crunch on Campus"[30] noted there has been a large increase in the utilization of so-called campus mental health services. The demand for appointments outpaces the supply, and budget caps are increasing. Most colleges and universities are trying

---

[30] http://www.wsj.com/news.us

to augment services. The need to do so has become more apparent as more students seek mental health care. This is good news since younger people seem to feel less stigma in seeking help.

In summary, youngsters don't appear with one illness, depression, in which antidepressants in some circumstances may have limited value. They may have early onset bipolar disorders, obsessive compulsive disorder, or ADHD for which expert pharmacotherapy may make a huge difference in their development and accomplishments.

Perhaps schools have been more aware of what are now identified as suicide clusters. There is a long list. MIT had six in 2014, and they were residents of the same dormitory. The College of William and Mary had several, and the University of Pennsylvania had a spate of suicides. One-third of schools do not have a psychiatrist available at all. The most important step a college or university can take to provide optimized evaluation and treatment for students is to hire a vetted brain psychiatrist who can provide expeditious and effective diagnostic services and pharmacological treatments for students with more serious illnesses. Every student seeking services should be administered the Mini International Neuropsychiatric Interview so lay therapists have the diagnostic data immediately available indicating medical (pharmacological) treatment is indicated. Would anything less be acceptable if the student had a subtler form of epilepsy like absence seizures? Would the school medical facilities skip the EEG?

One particularly ingenious approach to providing mental health services was recently originated by George Washington University. They opened a new wellness hub at the center of campus that combines mental health care, medical care, and health-promotion services in one location with the aim of minimizing the stigma of seeking professional help.

"Campus Suicide and the Pressure of Perfection"[31] focuses on the college environment. College counseling centers are finding more than half their clients have severe psychological problems. A number of professionals explain why.

---

[31] *The New York Times*, July 27, 2015 by Julie Scelfo.

Note the unfettered use of the treacherous dichotomy psychological problems. Students are under pressure to be effortlessly perfect, smart, accomplished, fit, beautiful, and popular—all without visible effort according to an investigative panel at the University of Pennsylvania. It even has a name, Penn Face, which is recognized as a potentially life-threatening aspect of campus culture. Similar studies at Duke University and Stanford reached similar conclusions.

Nobody should appear as if their struggling or unhappy. Small disappointments are reacted to as huge setbacks. Making mistakes is unacceptable. Even getting a B is categorized as being symbolic of failure. It is culturally necessary to measure up to one's peers, and they are viewed as talented and successful.

All this negative comparison is amplified by omnipresent social media that portrays successful, popular, and academically proficient students. One of the seniors said, "Nobody wants to be the one who is struggling while everyone else is doing great. Despite whatever's going on—if you're stressed, a bit depressed, if you're overwhelmed—you want to put up this positive front."

A number of professional campus therapists have had additional observations. The director of Penn's counseling services has observed a shift in how students react to challenges. They seem to magnify small setbacks into horrible mistakes. Another Penn counselor has noticed a similar change: getting a B can cause some students to fall apart.

A psychiatrist who practices as a member of the Penn faculty has observed the prevalence of shame, not being good enough, or being defective. Frank Bruni wrote *Where You Go Is Not Who You'll Be: An Antidote to College Admissions Mania.* The dean of freshman at Stanford, Julie Lythcott-Haims, over the years has observed a growing number of parents who show up on campus to help their offspring with just about everything: enrolling in classes, contacting professors, meeting with advisors. They keep in daily phone contact. Ms. Haims terms this *helicopter parenting* and pleads that children deserve to be strengthened and not strangled by the fierceness of a parent's love. She wrote *How to Raise an Adult: Break Free of the Overparenting Trap and Prepare Your Kid for Success.*

Psychologist Alice Miller wrote a book intended for therapists, *The Drama of the Gifted Child: The Search for the True Self,* which has been translated into thirty languages. She describes how intelligent and sensitive children, in particular, can become so attuned to parental expectations that they sacrifice their own needs and well-being to meet those expectations. In the process, they experience emotional emptiness and isolation. Depression is experienced as emptiness, futility, fear of impoverishment, and loneliness, which ultimately should be acknowledged as a tragic loss of self in childhood.

The book describes the experiences of two young women who matriculated at Penn. The first jumped to her death in her freshman year. The second young woman was stunned by the suicide. She did not personally know her, but she seemed popular, attractive, and talented. The second young woman, who will be termed Ms. X, set out from California after receiving her father's blessing: "The reason I'm living is to pass you off to your husband." Her father, an accomplished professional, was expressing his genuine hopes for his daughter. Penn is an Ivy League school, and students who matriculate there are generally in the higher echelons of academic achievement.

Ms. X decided, before her arrival on campus, that her main objectives were to major in mathematics, to become a teacher, to meet and marry a nice Christian boy, and settle down like her parents. Once on campus, she became aware of her fellow students. They seemed to have more drive and ability than she did. They seemed to have it all together. Their selfies seemed to sparkle with personality and amiability. She also became more aware of her attraction to cute girls, and she realized she was not heterosexual.

When she got a 60 percent in calculus course, she overheard an attractive young man making a snide remark about her. She felt more and more despondent, developing an overwhelming perspective that there was only one solution. She purchased razor blades and began cutting herself to prepare for the plan. Her goodbye letters were discovered by her roommate, and she was hospitalized. After lots of counseling, she was able to forge a new path for herself, confess her sexual feelings to her parents, and formulate more flexible academic and personal goals.

What is remarkable about this well-written article and its narration of Ms. X's personal history is the complete absence of reference to diagnosis (most likely MDD) and the treatment of the same—except for lots of counseling. Any impressionable younger person reading the article would never have the slightest idea there was an illness, major depressive disorder, that needed to be medically evaluated and diagnosed by a medically oriented psychiatrist (brain psychiatrist).

There is no brain there; it's all psychological treatment. It's as if a student had certain types of epilepsy that are not the more obvious grand mal type. Without seizures or psychomotor seizures, she managed with lots of counseling. This is a total and absolute demedicalization of the major psychiatric disorders. This occurs in frequent media portrayals of mental illnesses as just mental and psychological. The media really can't be held responsible for the trivialization and stigmatization of these serious brain disorders. It is psychiatry that perpetuates the demedicalization. The outcome is confusion and unnecessary suffering due to an absence of medically oriented brain psychiatrists in college communities. There is no serious consideration of the brain itself. This can only result in tragic therapeutic failures. And there was apparently a total absence of conceptualization of differential diagnosis: bipolar disorder, anxiety disorder, schizophrenia, hypothyroidism, hyperthyroidism, and so on! If undetected, each can result in disability or even death.

Crucial Elements of the History

History Component	Rationale
Psychiatric history	

Past psychiatric diagnosis and treatment	Allows confirmation of diagnosis and can guide treatment decisions.
Current suicidal thoughts and past suicide attempts	Crucial in assessing safety; past suicide attempts indicate increased risk of future attempts.
Substance abuse	Indicates contributing factors, such as alcohol use, for which additional intervention may be needed.
Problems with memory	Initial screen for cognitive problems and address with both patient and family if possible.
Medical history	
Presence of chronic pain	May exacerbate depression and indicate a need for additional treatment.
Polypharmacy	May complicate antidepressant treatment.
Problems with medication adherence	May lead to nonresponsive to antidepressant treatment.
Review of current medications	To identify any medications that may confer a predisposition to depression (propranolol, prednisone, etc.).
Social history	
Recent stressors or losses	Factors contributing to depression.
Available social support	Indicates extent of social engagement or isolation.
Access to transportation and the ability to drive	Indicates ability to engage socially and meet basic needs such as shopping for groceries.
Access to guns	Indicates increased risk that a suicide attempt would be lethal.

Family history	
Dementia	Indicates increased risk of dementia for the patient.
Suicide	Indicates increased risk of suicide for the patient.

In summary, youngsters just don't appear with one illness, depression, in which antidepressants would be the obvious option if symptoms are severe. They may have early onset bipolar disorders, obsessive-compulsive disorder, or ADHD. Expert pharmacotherapy may make a huge difference in their development and accomplishments, and antidepressant use alone may be contraindicated.

GLOSSARY

brain structures associated with symptoms. Posterior cortex, anterior and midline structures, the amygdalae and associated network including dorsolateral-prefrontal cortex, nucleus accumbens. Reduced functional capacity. Inadequate regulation of emotional and cognitive responses.

calcium (between and inside neurons). Levels increased in bipolar disorder.

calcium dysfunction. Affects development of brain. Causes neurons to migrate differently.

gene expression. Altered in bipolar disorder. Causes excessive manufacture of receptors and ion channels in neurons and excessive calcium signaling.

ion channel. Permits ions to enter and leave neuron, for example, calcium, for which there is increased turnover in bipolar disorder.

receptor. In membrane of neuron upon which neurotransmitters dock, causing passage of signal into the interior of the cell.

stem cells. Through specialized laboratory techniques, skin cells are taken back to primitive early stage and then reprogrammed as neurons.

white matter. Especially uncinate fasciculus. Loss of integrity. Altered signaling in bipolar disorder.

CHAPTER 13

Bipolar Disorder

Bipolar disorder is not some wisp of a mental health problem as if all one had to do is floss more mentally, so to speak, to overcome it. Psychiatry, however, by including it as a mental problem in its diagnostic manual, trivializes it in the same manner as severe major depression. In many instances, the disease attacks and destroys the dreams and lives of those afflicted with it. It leaves the sufferer totally at the mercy of emotional storms not controllable by the strongest will, which are generated by violent dysregulation of the physical brain. The main pharmacological agents, which attempt to deintensify symptoms, are, for the most part, identical to the anticonvulsants prescribed by neurologists to treat grand mal epilepsy and other forms of seizure disorders. Like many neurological illnesses, such as epilepsy and multiple sclerosis, it shaves seven to ten years off the life span on average. And overlaying the symptoms and disabilities of the disease itself is the suffocating fog of being labeled mental, which the neurological disorders escape.

Dr. Kay Redfield Jamison is a professor of psychology at the Johns Hopkins University School of Medicine. In 1990, she and Frederik Goodwin, MD, coauthored and published the authoritative textbook on bipolar disorder. She has written more than one hundred articles on the disorder as well as several books for lay people, including *An Unquiet Mind* (1999) an autobiography detailing her personal struggle with the disease. In "A Psychologist's Career-Altering Mental Illness,"[32] she describes the onset of her own symptoms in adolescence.

Out of the blue, she had spells of being unable to get out of bed and just wanting to die. She could not concentrate even to read. These symptoms originally caused career-related difficulties. Finally, when she was already a psychologist, she was fortunate enough to be diagnosed accurately and was started on lithium. It was still difficult for her to accept or fully comprehend her illness because she discontinued the lithium, and then she attempted suicide in the midst of a severe clinical depression. At that point, she became serious about understanding her own illness, and she has gone on to an illustrious career.

Her new insight permitted her to comprehend her father's symptoms. He was an air force officer with alcohol problems and severe mood episodes. She sent him a copy of *An Unquiet Mind,* and he was able to transform the course of his own disease by accepting treatment. Upon reflecting on her father's side of the family, it was evident other relatives also had been bipolar. She felt that going public with her illness allowed her to reach out in a personal way to other sufferers.

Noticeable in Dr. Jamison and her father's personal histories are the extended periods of symptoms, suffering, and disabilities before the diagnosis of bipolar disorder was considered. She notes how important it is that providers become familiar with the illness and how to diagnose and treat it, which requires in-depth knowledge and skill in pharmacological treatment to control it.

Unfortunately, the current so-called mental health system—with rare exceptions and on an unpredictable basis—is tragically scattershot in identifying practitioners with the required training. Years or decades can pass with cumulative symptoms and disabilities growing before a patient meets up with a skilled practitioner. It's as if a neurology patient with atypical seizures runs from physical therapist to physical therapist without ever being evaluated and diagnosed by

---

[32] Avis-Thomas-Lester, December 16, 2009, *The Washington Post.*

a neurologist trained and experienced in diagnosing and prescribing appropriately complex pharmacology for the varieties of seizure disorders.

What can one say about individuals who display the following behaviors? Surely they are mentally ill! The behaviors do not occur in all individuals, but most have two, three, or more: becoming, for no particular reason, irritable, hostile, fatigued, or depressed. Having insomnia. Abusing illicit drugs, alcohol, marijuana, stimulants, cocaine, and opioids. Wearing unusual accoutrements such as pierced rings in unusual parts of the body: the tongue, nipples, navel, or external genitalia. Sporting multiple tattoos. Wearing flamboyantly colored clothes. Engaging in excessive and unusual sexual activity. Dating several individuals on the same day and having sex. Having relations with one's spouse and also visiting prostitutes. Compulsively masturbating. There is often a history of educational, vocational, and marital instability. Not obtaining a degree, losing and/or switching jobs, having multiple marriages and divorces. Surely one most conclude such individuals are obviously mentally ill!

At the University of Michigan Medical School,[33] Professor Sue O'Shea, PhD, and her staff asked themselves what makes a person subject to such excessive behaviors, manic highs, and deep depressed lows? Why does bipolar disorder run so strongly in families even though no single gene is causative?

Employing sophisticated laboratory techniques, researchers scraped skin cells from patients with bipolar disorder, converted them into pluripotent stem cells (iPSCs), which are present in very early embryonic development and have the capacity to develop into the major different tissues and organs in the adult body. They were then able to transition the stem cells into neurons of the brain for patients with and without bipolar disorders.

When they compared the neurons from each group, the neurons from bipolar patients behaved differently than those from nonaffected

---

[33] "First Stem Cell Study of Bipolar Disorder," *Translational Psychiatry*, March 25, 2014.

individuals. There was much greater gene expression for membrane receptors and ion channels, resulting in much greater signaling with calcium between cells and increased amounts of calcium inside the neurons. There was evidence calcium dysfunction also affects development of the embryonic brain, causing neurons to migrate differently.

The administration of lithium normalized the calcium-derived abnormalities of the neurons. They concluded it was evidence for a genetic causation of bipolar disorder.[34] They determined the critical brain structures responsible for the symptoms were the dorsolateral prefrontal cortex, components of the limbic system and basal ganglia, and a white matter tract, the uncinate fascicules. (The prefrontal cortex is divided into three parts, dorsolateral (DLPFC), ventrolateral, and orbitofrontal.) The limbic system, in the center of the brain, has several important substructures: the hypothalamus, thalamus, cingulate gyrus, parahippocampal gyrus, and hippocampus. The basal ganglia are active in the planning and coordination of movement and play a role in behavioral responses. The uncinate fascicules is a major white matter tract serving as a cable to connect the above structures to one another so electrical and chemical messages are passed between them efficiently. White matter tracts are often defective in bipolar disorder.

Dr. Radaelli considers bipolar disorder to be a severe, disabling, life-threatening disease, which through underlying disturbances in emotional regulation and distortions of thinking results in serious dysfunctions in memory, attention, judgment, decision-making, and social interaction. His group studied fifty-two patients with the disease and forty unaffected individuals. They utilized detailed neuropsychological testing and imaging studies (functional MRI, positron emission tomography, and single-photon-emission computerized tomography).

They identified the DLPFC, the nucleus accumbens, and the

---

[34] Researcher D. Radacli, et al., The Department of Clinical Neurosciences at the Instituto Scientifico Ospedale San Raffoele, Milan, Italy www.sciencedirect.com, May 19, 2014.

amygdalae as making up network crucial for regulation of mood, emotions, and elements of thinking. They found that individuals with bipolar disorder have reduced functional connectivity in this network, resulting in inadequate regulation of emotional and cognitive responses. These abnormalities are also associated with a loss of white matter integrity, particularly the uncinate fasciculus.

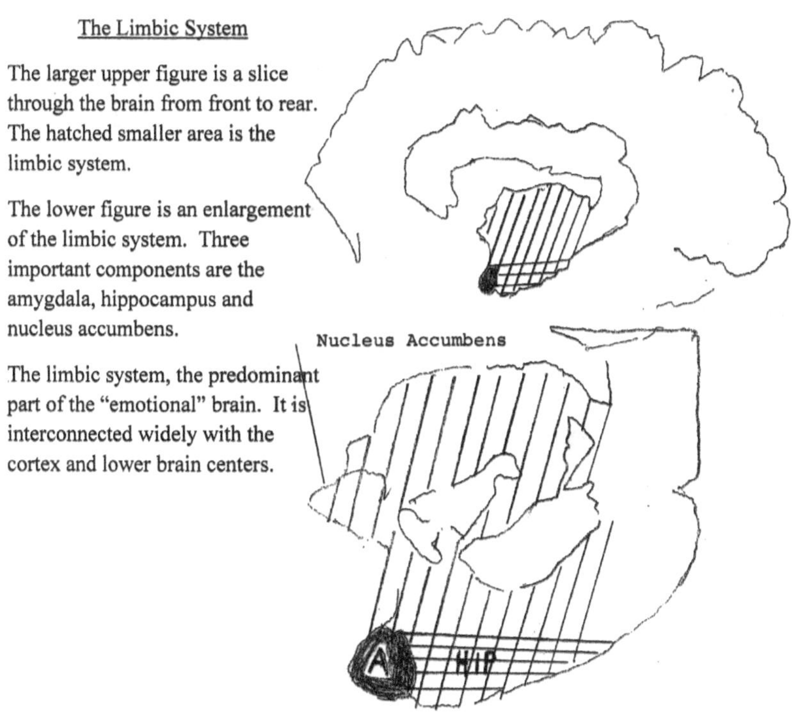

The Limbic System

Neuroimaging methods also are promising to differentiate unipolar from bipolar spectrum major depressive episodes.[35] The posterior

[35] "Differences in Functional Connectivity in Major Depression versus Bipolar II Depression," Marchand, J. et al. *Journal of Affective Disorders*, February 20, 2013.

cingulate cortex, an important brain region having functional connectivity to various brain networks of the anterior and posterior midline cortex, and the amygdalae in bipolar disorder may function defectively, resulting in increases in negative emotions and thinking distortions such as intense self-referential ideations (beliefs others are thinking harshly about oneself in the absence of actual evidence).

Anticonvulsants

Specialized physicians, neurologists, treat a variety of seizure disorders with anticonvulsants. Certainly, there is no question in this modern era that epilepsy is a physical disease of the brain and anticonvulsants are an appropriate physical treatment. In the modern era, anticonvulsants are also prescribed for the treatment of bipolar spectrum disorders, which are still classified by psychiatry as a mental health problem. Anticonvulsant medications magically transform from physical treatments for epilepsy to mental treatments for bipolar illnesses. In the process, those suffering from the latter experience the symptoms and disabilities of the illness—and the stigmatization of psychiatry labeling them mentally ill.

GLOSSARY

agonist. A neurotransmitter that turns on its receptor.

benzodiazepines. A class of psychoactive drugs that enhances the actions of the neurotransmitter gamma-aminobutyric acid (GABA) at the GABA-A receptor, resulting in antianxiety action. If given in excess, they may promote excessive sedation. Individuals with addictive disease may abuse them. Examples are Xanax, Ativan, Klonopin and Valium (brand names).

beta-blockers. A class of drugs used to manage cardiac arrhythmias and hypertension. They are antagonists to adrenaline and noradrenaline at adrenergic beta receptors. In certain instances, they serve as antianxiety medication.

buspirone. An antianxiety medication used to treat anxiety disorders—but not panic disorder. Unlike benzodiazepines, it has a delayed period of onset, but is not habit-forming.

cyclosporine. An amino acid derivative used to treat tuberculosis. It may have antianxiety properties and diminish addictive urges.

EKG. Electrocardiogram.

endocannabinoid system. A group of endogenous (present in the brain) receptors involved in appetite, pain sensation, mood, and memory.

endogenous. Substances and processes originating from within the organism itself.

executive planning. A set of cognitive processes including attentional control, inhibitory control, working memory, and reasoning ability.

GABA-A receptor. It binds gamma-amino-butyric acid, the major inhibitory neurotransmitter in the nervous system.

GABA-B receptor agonist. A drug that stimulates one or more GABA receptors, in this case, the GABA-B receptor. GABA receptors may play a role in the symptoms of MDD and its treatment.

glucocorticoid receptors. They bind the stress hormone cortisol.

glutamatergic-N-methyl-D-aspartate receptor (NMDAr). A glutamate receptor activated by glutamate and glycine. It is affected by many psychoactive drugs as well as drugs of abuse like ketamine, phencyclidine, and alcohol. Hypofunction is a main contributor to symptoms, particularly in schizophrenia. Ketamine and phencyclidine can evoke all the symptoms of schizophrenia through powerful antagonistic actions at NMDAr.

hyperarousal symptoms. When the autonomic (sympathetic) nervous system is in an excessive state of activation, which is often associated with symptomatic anxiety, insomnia, difficulty concentrating, fatigue, irritability, and extreme vigilance.

hypothalamic-pituitary-adrenal axis (HPA). A complex of three endocrine glands: the adrenal, pituitary, and hypothalamus. It produces steroid hormones and is involved in a complex interplay. It controls reactions to stress and regulates digestion, the immune system, mood, emotions, sexuality, and energy storage and expenditure.

MAOI. A type of antidepressant including Marplan, Ensam, Nardil, and Parnate (brand names) that may have efficacy if other antidepressants fail. Prescriber, however, must have experience in their prescription since very serious side effects are possible.

neuromodulator. A physiological process in which a given neuron uses one or more chemicals to regulate diverse populations of neurons.

oxytocin. A neuropeptide hormone used in obstetrics to increase the speed of labor. It has acquired the nickname "the love hormone."

partial agonist. A neurotransmitter that partly turns on a receptor.

presynaptic alpha 2 adrenergic inhibitory autoreceptor. They play an essential role in regulating neurotransmitter release from sympathetic nerves and adrenergic neurons.

presynaptic serotonin 5-HT1A receptor. A subtype of serotonin receptor that binds serotonin, which is widespread. Some actions include decreasing impulsivity and aggression, improving sociability, and reduction in illicit drug-seeking behavior.

postsynaptic alpha-adrenergic blocker (antagonist). It inhibits the release of noradrenaline, which reduces blood pressure and anxiety.

postsynaptic 5-HT2 and 5-HT3 receptors. The blockade of 5-HT2 may facilitate the efficacy of SSRI antidepressants. Agonists of 5-HT3 reduce nausea and vomiting.

QT prolongation on the EKG. Involving the QT interval, which represents the contraction of the ventricles of the heart. The prescriber must be aware if any drugs prescribed will prolong the interval, which could result in a fatal cardiac arrhythmia.

serotonin receptors. There is a quite a variety, some of which have subtypes. Examples of serotonin receptors are 5-HT1, 5-HT2, 5-HT3, 5-HT4, 5-HT5, 5-HT6, and 5-HT7.

tricyclic antidepressant. Among the earliest antidepressants developed and may have efficacy if newer antidepressants fail. The prescriber must be familiar with ordering laboratory levels of the tricyclic and have knowledge of possibly dangerous EKG (electrocardiogram) abnormalities.

ventricular arrhythmias. This can be caused if a drug or drugs sufficiently prolong the QT interval, causing arrhythmia, which is often fatal.

CHAPTER 14

Veterans

The Vietnam veteran presented himself in the office of this author for the initial evaluation. He had such a flat-looking facial expression. He spoke in a dull monotone. His movements seemed retarded—as if he was depleted of energy. He cast his eyes downward. There was a complete absence of life force, a joyless effect, a saddened mood, a 180-degree opposite of any hint of enthusiasm or joie de vivre. A gray-dark world seemed to emanate from his very countenance.

During the evaluation, it became apparent that life held no meaning for him. He looked forward to nothing. His existence was a perpetual numbness. He really did not want to exist any longer. If not for his faith, he would have committed suicide! Even his feelings toward God were deeply conflicted. While realizing suicide would jeopardize his soul, he knew he needed God. However, it became apparent that he was enraged at God because of his suffering!

He went through the agony of flashbacks, even while awake, becoming submerged as if he were still in combat. Shells swished overhead, and his buddy was instantly decapitated. For several nights after such flashbacks, he couldn't sleep, he was agitated, he couldn't relax for an instant, and he'd become exhausted, fatigued, and totally depleted. He'd be frazzled, experience uncontrolled ruminations and anxieties, and remain in a cocoon of hopelessness.

He was living alone. His wife had left. Even if she had been supportive, he was devoid of the capacity to accept or respond to her support. This veteran had severe post-traumatic stress disorder. Did he have a mental illness a mental health problem? All he has to do was just decide to pull himself up and get over it! Psychiatry is labeling him mentally ill. That is what psychiatry has always done and continues to do. Psychiatry wants to add a second layer to his suffering by stigmatizing him, humiliating him, and accusing him of being mental!

Post-traumatic stress disorder is not a mental problem. It is a physical brain disease with some mental symptoms. The mental symptoms can arise from a number of body organs—the thyroid, the adrenal gland, the parathyroids—neurological illnesses of the brain, from systemic symptoms, fever, low or high blood sugar, and other causes.

The Vietnam War

Post-traumatic stress disorder entered the national consciousness when many Vietnam veterans showed symptoms of the illness: vivid flashbacks of combat in which they actually believed they were back in actual combat, crushing anxiety, and terror. These acute episodic symptoms occurred in the context of continuous emotional numbness, avoidance of social activities, anhedonia (inability to obtain enjoyment or be interested in or obtain pleasure from activities previously rewarding), impaired capacity to maintain relationships, insomnia, irritability, and loneliness.

Of the 2.6 million men who served within the borders of Vietnam, approximately 1.4 million were directly involved in combat or exposed to enemy attack. A total of 58,202 died (47,378 directly from hostile action), 303,704 were wounded, and 153,329 were hospitalized for same, and 75,000 were disabled—23,214 with 100 percent disability—5,283 lost a limb, and 1,081 sustained multiple amputations. Amputation or crippling wounds to the lower extremities were 300 percent higher than in World War II. Multiple amputations occurred at the rate of 18.4 percent compared to 5.7 percent in WWII.

The National Vietnam Veterans Longitudinal Study (NVVLS) was mandated by Congress to determine the prevalence, course, and associated illnesses of war-zone post-traumatic stress disorders across a twenty-five-year period. The researchers studied a representative national sample of 2,348 veterans who served in war zones. The study was conducted from July 2012 until May 2013. Forty years after the war ended, 20 percent had died, and 4.5 percent still had full blown PTSD, severe chronicity, and disability. An additional 10 percent had subthreshold PTSD, which can also be associated with suffering and disability. Of those still ill after forty years, twice as many had deteriorated as had improved. In addition, as they aged, the symptoms and disabilities of PTSD were complicated by the stresses of aging, chronic illnesses, declining social support, cognitive deterioration, and the distress of unwanted memories.

Less attention has been paid to female veterans. Although not directly engaged in combat, they still had a wide range of military experiences. They were exposed to casualties, accidents, interpersonal violence, and sometimes sexual harassment; 16 percent still had symptoms of full-blown PTSD decades after military service.

In a recent study in *Circulation,* fifty thousand female nurses had their health tracked for twenty years.[36] They were evaluated for symptoms of PTSD: staying away from places or activities that are a reminder of a previous traumatic event, loss of interest in previously important enjoyable activities, finding it hard to feel love or affection, and becoming jumpy or easily startled by ordinary noises or movements. The women with PTSD had a 60 percent higher incidence of cerebral-vascular disease, heart attacks, and strokes, which also occurred at much younger ages in comparison to women without PTSD.

---

[36] June 29, 2015, conducted by Jennifer Sumnes et al. from the Columbia University Mailman School of Public Health in NYC.

With veterans, wouldn't it be kinder and more rational to lift the burden of being labeled as mental cases? Are they really mental? Haven't they suffered enough without this additional shroud of stigmatization and humiliation being cast over them by psychiatry?

GLOSSARY

anterior cingulate cortex. The frontal part of the cingulate cortex plays a role in cognition and emotion

cingulate gyrus. Important part of limbic system that regulates emotion and pain.

corticostriatal-thalamic-cortical circuit. Dysregulated feedback loop in OCD.

limbic system. A set of brain structures buried under the cortex and involved in emotions and motivations.

orbital frontal cortex. A prefrontal cortex region involved in cognitive processing and decision-making.

ventral internal capsule. Carries a large number of motor and sensory fibers to and from the cortex.

ventral striatum. Important for reward system.

CHAPTER 15

OCD

Why would anyone choose to spend their time as the following woman does? Why doesn't she just snap out of it? After all, it's just a mental problem. She's either weak-willed or stupid!

Gloria remembers not feeling well starting at age five. She developed anxiety, fears, and rituals, including excessive hand washing to counteract fear of the devil. The symptoms were quite intense. She was very ashamed of her symptoms and hid them from her parents for a number of years. She remembers being intensely lonely from the age of five onward. Looking back over her life at the age of forty-five, she has deeply regretted not having a career or a romantic relationship. It could be said, unfortunately, that dealing with her OCD has been her career, consuming great increments of her time and energy for decades. Her illness would be classified as a lifelong one.

Her day begins at noon when she gets up. She has a part-time job in the early afternoon caring for a mentally retarded person for about two hours. When she arrives back to her apartment at approximately three o'clock, she begins her routine of strenuous extensive regimented exercising for two or more hours, driven by a belief that she has no right to relax or enjoy herself unless she does so. Soon after, she begins hours of time-consuming rituals around preparation of and then consuming an evening meal. Her rituals are so intricate and complex that she has significantly reduced her caloric intake. She rarely weighs more than ninety pounds (she is five foot five) and often requires acute medical management when her weight drops to eighty-two or eighty-three pounds or her electrolytes become abnormal. She requires emergency hospitalization when her sodium drops to critically low levels.

She finally completes her entire supper routine at around ten. After a small break, she begins a regime of extensive mental rituals, hours-long repetition of prayers, and reviewing lists and phrases in a stereotyped way. Finally, close to five o'clock, she gets into bed. Possibly, as a benefit of medication, there has been a reduction in her terrifying preoccupation she will come to grievous harm—by going to hell—if she did not perform another extensive set of rituals.

OCD is such a complex, multisymptomatic illness. There is a large set of symptoms she did not personally have, but which can occur: contamination concerns, washing compulsions, extensive hand washing, checking compulsions, preoccupation with symmetry and order, intrusive images or urges of harming other individuals (though such impulses are rarely acted out), tics, trichotillomania, hoarding, body dimorphic disorder, or often in association with OCD, bulimia, or self-injury.

Since high school, she has had a continuous roster of treatments, general psychotherapies, specialized therapy for OCD, and several hospitalizations. Unfortunately, she hasn't been motivated or possibly is unable to utilize the most specific therapy for OCD: response-prevention therapy. She, over the years, has been on a number of medications: clomipramine and then tryptophan with some benefit, fluoxetine, sertraline, clomipramine again, then escitalopram added to it. More recently, she has had minor improvement on high-dose Anafranil combined with escitalopram. High-dose Anafranil requires careful medical supervision, including periodic blood levels to prevent elevations that could induce seizures.

She agreed to have a consultation with a specialist in OCD in another state who suggested sequential augmentations with two glutamate modulators (rilozole and memantine), the serotonin 5HT-3 antagonist, ondansetron, and the synthetic opiate tramadol. In addition to specialized psychotherapy and complex psychopharmacology, neurosurgery can reduce OCD symptoms, but she is too fearful to consider it.

What is pitiful is the additional suffering, stigmatization, and humiliation stemming from psychiatry's continued classification of OCD as a mental health problem.

Howard Robert Hughes Jr. was enormously successful in multiple varied endeavors, and he was a celebrity who had a fatal character flaw. In spite of his financial successes, and in the absence of any terminal physical illness like cancer, he became unimaginably debilitated. Although his natural height was six feet four inches, he weighed only ninety-three pounds, a long skeleton over which was draped a canopy of ghostlike, pallid skin.[37] His fingernails and toenails grotesquely protruded to the point of being many inches long and curling back on themselves. He would not let anyone touch him. He rented the entire top floor of the Acapulco Princess Hotel.[38] Two personal physicians were in attendance, residing in a room adjoining the penthouse.

Members of his personal staff took special alarm as Hughes appeared to pass into a delirious state. They summoned a third physician who arrived early the next day. Also, a fourth physician, a Mexican, recommended he not be hospitalized in Mexico, and be flown back to the United States. His staff busily began researching medical centers for the best option. They decided on the University of Texas Medical Center in Houston. He was transported to the airport and taken into one of his own aircraft. His white jet took off and rose sharply over the Sierra Madre mountains. Below were Mexico's jagged peaks, lush forests, and sun-bleached villages white against green hills. It was a perfect day for flying, the kind of day Howard

---

[37] "Howard Hughes' Doctor Gives Chilling Description of his Strange Patient's Final Hours," Time Inc. Network, July 30, 1979, Vol. 12 No. 5, by Dennis Breo.
[38] *Howard Hughes: His Life and Madness.* D. L. Barlett and James B. Steele, 1979. W. W. Norton.

Hughes would have loved to be at the controls.[39] Before they reached Houston, he seemed to be fading into a coma. His pulse weakened, and then his breathing stopped. He had finally come home to Texas as a cachectic corpse. Who was this man who through lack of will couldn't conquer his OCD, which according to psychiatry, is just a mental health problem?

He was born Dec. 24, 1905[40] in either Humble or Houston. His mother died when he was seventeen, and his father died less than two years later. He inherited 75 percent of the family fortune, and on his nineteenth birthday, he was declared an emancipated minor. From an early age, he became an excellent golfer and played with top national players. He quit to take up other interests and situated himself in Los Angeles to produce motion pictures. His first two films, *Everybody's Acting* (1927) and *Two Arabian Knights* (1928) actually made money, the latter winning the first Academy Award for best director of a comedy picture. Two additional films were nominated for Academy Awards. A fifth film *Hell's Angels* (1930) received an Academy Award for best cinematography. He made $8 million profit on it. A 1943 film *The Outlaw* featured leading lady Jane Russell, for whom he designed a special brassiere, which she declined to wear. In 1948, he gained control of RKO, a major motion production company in Hollywood which included RKO pictures, RKO studios, RKO Theatres (a large chain of movie theatres), the RKO Radio Network (a network of radio stations), selling it six months later to the General Tire and Rubber Company, making $6.5 million in personal profit.

He dated many of the most famous actresses of the era—Bette Davis, Ava Gardner, Olivia de Havilland, Katherine Hepburn, and Gene Tierney.

Tierney said, "I don't think Howard could love anything that did not have a motor in it."

In 1932, he founded Hughes Aircraft Company in a rented corner of a Lockheed Aircraft Corporation hangar in Burbank, California.

---

[39] Ibid, 24–25.

[40] Howard Hughes, from Wikipedia, the free encyclopedia.

During World War II, he built it into a major defense contractor. After the war, it was a major player in defense manufacturing, including spacecraft vehicles, military aircraft, radar systems, electro-optical systems, the first working laser, aircraft computer systems, missile systems, ion-propulsion engines for space travel, and commercial satellites. Ultimately, Hughes donated all the stock of his companies in the aviation and space industries to the Howard Hughes Medical Institute.

In 1939, Hughes bought $7 million of Trans World Airlines (TWA) stock, which he sold in 1966 for $547 million. In 1970, he went back into the airline business, acquiring San Francisco-based Air West Airlines, which subsequently was acquired by Republic Airlines, which eventually merged into Delta Airlines, now one of the largest in the world.

In the 1930s, in addition to designing and manufacturing planes, he set many world records as a pilot, including a new transcontinental airspeed record in 1937, flying nonstop from Los Angeles to Newark in seven hours and twenty-eight minutes, and in July 1938, completing a flight around the world in three days and nineteen hours. Afterward, he received a ticker-tape parade in Manhattan. He received a special Congressional Gold Medal in 1939 in recognition of his contributions to the science of aviation.

In 1953, Hughes launched the Howard Hughes Medical Institute, located in Chevy Chase, Maryland, with the expressed goal of furthering basic biomedical research. He was the major contributor to its funding. As of 2007, it was the largest private organization devoted to biological and medical research with an endowment of $16.3 billion.

From 1966 to 1976, accompanied by his entourage of personal aides and physicians, he began moving from one hotel to another in many different cities. In 1966, one of the hotels he stayed at, the Desert Inn in Las Vegas, began insisting he move out because he was refusing to leave. He resolved the conflict by buying the hotel and then branching out, purchasing several hotel-casinos in Las Vegas, including the Castaways, New Frontier, the Landmark Hotel and Casino, and the Sands. When the trademark neon light of the small Silver Slipper Casino across from his room kept him up at night, he purchased that casino also. While he was in a purchasing mood, he also acquired several local television stations. He had a taste for ice cream. On one occasion, he ordered his staff to bring him Baskin-Robbins banana nut ice cream. They learned that Baskin-Robbins had discontinued the flavor for ordinary commercial use, but they agreed to make a special batch of two hundred gallons for Hughes. When the ice cream arrived, Hughes announced he no longer had a taste for that flavor, insisting on only chocolate marshmallow. Reportedly, the hotel ended up distributing free banana nut ice cream to its casino customers for over a year.

Hughes had two nearly fatal crashes, one in 1943 and the other in 1946. In the second crash, the plane destroyed three houses, and the fuel tanks exploded. He managed to pull himself out of the flaming wreckage, sustaining a crushed collarbone, multiple cracked ribs, a crushed chest, a collapsed left lung that shifted his heart to the right side of his chest cavity, and numerous third-degree burns. As he lay in his hospital bed, he was happy that his mind was still intact. He decided he did not like the design of his particular hospital bed and designed a customized bed with hot and cold running water and independently moving sections operated by thirty electric motors. He never got to use it, but some of its features were incorporated into current hospital beds. His physicians felt his recovery was nearly miraculous. Hughes believed his recovery was not due to modern medicine but freshly squeezed orange juice, which he personally witnessed being squeezed each day. It is probable his addiction to codeine used as a painkiller started then.

When he died in 1976, his estate was valued at $2.5 billion. Evidently, his OCD became symptomatic in his late twenties or early thirties. Close friends reported he was obsessed with the size of the peas, one at his favorite vegetables, using a special fork to sort them by size. During the filming of *The Outlaw* in 1943, he became fixated on the fabric of Jane Russell's blouse. When the fabric bunched up, it gave the appearance of having two nipples on each breast.

His most extreme obsession was preventing germs from coming near him. As his illness progressed, he took complicated precautions. Doors and windows were sealed with masking tape. The aides who worked with him daily were required to follow a set of carefully prescribed rituals. They handed him papers or objects wrapped in "paddles" or layers of Kleenex. They spread "insulation," or layers of paper towels on his bed, chair, and bathroom floor. They guarded against the delivery of mail sent by someone he feared had been exposed to contagious germs.

One can only imagine his personal anxiety and torment! During his final decade, when he was living in a series of hotel penthouses, he remained in darkened rooms, lying naked, often watching serial movies. According to his aides, *Ice Station Zebra* was spliced so it ran on a continuous loop—and he viewed more than 150 times. He refused to have his hair cut, beard trimmed, or nails clipped. The OCD transitioned to a psychotic state punctuated by codeine addition via self-administered injections several times daily, culminating in his tragic death.

Mr. Hughes never received treatment for the OCD or the codeine dependence. It is impossible to imagine he would even have accepted the label mentally ill. It is possible, if he was told he had a brain illness, a physical illness, and had the very concept mental illness had not existed, he could have been more open to receiving treatment. This issue persists up to the present. How many thousands turn away from treatment to avoid the humiliation and stigmatization of the mental illness label perpetuated by psychiatry?

How can it be that a mental problem can improve after neurosurgery on selected regions of the brain? The neurosurgeons must be slicing out unconscious aggressive urges and sexual impulses, thereby relieving the patients of all these deep, painful psychoanalytic mental conflicts.

Neurosurgical procedures used to treat physical diseases in

neurology, tumors, abnormal seizure foci, etc., when similarly used to treat so-called mental illness, must transform into hocus-pocus mental treatments to alleviate mental health problems.

Neurosurgical procedures have been controversial in the treatment of psychiatric disorders. In the past, techniques were poorly researched, did not follow rigorous designs and formats, had poor follow-up, and had untoward ill effects. This has dramatically changed for the better with modern neuroscience and imaging technology, refinement of neurosurgical techniques, and systemic selection and follow-up with patients.

Surgical interventions may be considered for patients with severe MDD and OCD who have not responded to the traditional treatments and who remain severely symptomatic and disabled. In specialized treatment centers, multidisciplinary teams consisting of psychiatrists, neurosurgeons, psychologists, and other specialists carefully review each case, establish that conventional treatment has indeed failed, and determine that neurosurgical treatment may be beneficial.

Modern neurosurgical approaches employ a high level of precision, permitting precise targeting of troublesome brain circuits by employing stereotaxic methodology. Modern computer-based imaging techniques permit localization of dysfunctional brain areas smaller than a millimeter. DBS (deep-brain stimulation) is used to treat Parkinson's disease, MDD, and OCD.

In the largest study of DBS and MDD, fifteen severely ill patients underwent bilateral DBS electrode implantation in the ventral internal capsule/ventral striatum. After twelve months, more than half showed long-term improvement in depression severity, quality of life, and short-term memory. Safety outcomes were good. Patients with incapacitating OCD show a similar level of improvement.

There are four different neurosurgical operations used to treat severe disabling MDD and OCD: cingulotomy, capsulotomy, subcaudate tractomy, and limbic leucotomy. The most frequently used procedure is the cingulotomy. The cingulate gyrus is critical in cortico-striatal-thalamic pathways in mediating the transfer of information from the anterior cingulate cortex to the orbital frontal cortex and the limbic system. In the cingulate, the anterior portion of the cingulate gyrus is interrupted, which reduces communication between it and the frontal lobes.

In a recent prospective study, forty-four patients with severe OCD were followed from before treatment to six months post-surgery. Nearly 50 percent showed significant improvement. Cosgrove, a researcher at Massachusetts General Hospital in Boston reported on the safety of more than eight hundred cingulotomies over a forty-year period at that hospital. There were no deaths and only two infections. Response rates were high (68 percent).

When will these neurosurgically treated patients labeled as mentally ill by psychiatry escape the specter of shame, stigmatization, and humiliation inflicted by the dark label of mental illness?

GLOSSARY

acetylcholinergic receptor (a7). A very important receptor associated with cognitive deficits in schizophrenia.

apoptosis. A built-in program of neurons, which if triggered by certain conditions, causes the neuron to destroy itself.

auditory cortex. Part of the temporal lobe that processes auditory information.

BDNF. A neurotrophic factor sustaining neuron health.

dentate gyrus. Part of the hippocampus. Contributes to the formation of new episodic memories and the spontaneous exploration of novel environments.

dendrites, dendritic spines. Dendrites are filament-type structures protruding from the bodies of neurons upon which are numerous protrusions to which the axons of other neurons attach.

dopamine. One of the important neuroamine neurotransmitters with extensive actions in the brain, particularly the reward systems.

epigenetic mechanisms. Heritable alterations not due to changes in DNA sequence, but methyl group tags and histone modification.

extra-pyramidal symptoms. Particular symptoms caused by Parkinson's disease (tremor, muscle stiffness, retardation of movement) or as a side effect, particularly to first-generation antipsychotics.

frontal lobes. One of four major lobes of the cortex controlling cognitive skills, problem-solving, memory, language, and judgment. In essence, the control panel of our personality.

free radicals. Organic molecules that cause damage to normal tissue and are associated with disease and aging. Examples include chlorofluocarbons, ultraviolet radiation, and molecules with an unpaired electron.

GABAergic neurotransmission. Nerve impulses set off when GABA lands on its designated receptors on a neuron's membrane.

gene coding. Areas of genes associated with specific products. For example, the genes that code for the digestive hormone, insulin.

glial cells. They closely accompany neurons and provide for their optimal functioning.

glutaminergic neurotransmission. The nerve signals set off when the neurotransmitter, glutamate, binds to its specific receptors.

glutathione. A substance produced in the liver involved in many body processes, including building tissue by making required chemicals and proteins for the immune system.

hippocampus. The part of brain involved in memory formation and memory storage. It is part of limbic system.

hypoxia. When tissues do not receive sufficient oxygen to maintain normal cell processes, resulting in cell dysfunction or death.

hypothalamus. A section of the brain responsible for the production of many hormones. It links the nervous system to the endocrine system via the pituitary gland.

midbrain. A portion of the brain associated with vision, hearing, motor control, sleep/wake, arousal (alertness), and temperature regulation.

mitochondria. An organelle (entity found within a cell body). It has a double membrane and generates the energy required for cell processes with the molecule adenosine triphosphate (ATP).

mitosis abnormality. An essential process in the accurate division of a cell into two duplicates. A number of situations lead to errors that can result in malformations. Good health habits are preventative.

MRI, MRS, DTI. Medical-imaging techniques used to visualize the anatomy and physiological processes of diseases.

myelin fibers. Of nerves, having a protective myelin sheath or covering.

negative symptoms. Symptoms of schizophrenia that degrade the capacity for normal social interaction. Social withdrawal, flat affect, reduced speech.

neurogenesis. Process by which neurons are generated from neural stem cells.

neuroplasticity. The brain's capacity to adapt and reorganize itself, allowing compensation for damage caused by injury or disease.

neurotrophic factors. A family of biomolecules that are peptides or small proteins and support neuron health.

oxidative stress. When there is an excess of free radicals (molecules with an unpaired electron) that the body is unable to neutralize, causing tissue damage.

parietal cortex. One of the four major lobes. Its main responsibility is processing sensory information.

pharmacodynamics/pharmacokinetics. The first is the study of the effects of a drug on the body. The second is the effect the body has on the drug.

positive symptoms. Reference to psychotic symptoms that are quite apparent to an observer, such as hallucinations and/or delusions.

prodromal phase. The early symptomatic phase of a disease when milder symptoms are occurring, but not yet full-blown symptoms.

risk gene. A particular version of a gene that may predispose to a disease, i.e., BRCA gene and breast cancer.

stem cell. Primitive undifferentiated cells that can differentiate into specialized cells.

striatal region, striatum. A critical component of reward system, it is the primary input into basal ganglia.

vivo (in vivo). Studies or experiments performed on living organisms.

CHAPTER 16

Schizophrenia

She is obviously very intelligent, and quite capable academically. Why didn't she just snap out of her mental problems and get on with her studies? Is there some characterological or moral weakness that explains her lack of responsibility for herself?

She was a law student at the University of Oxford in England. She developed the belief her thoughts had killed thousands of people. She also saw a huge spider crawling up her wall. She was hospitalized. She lost behavioral control and was placed in restraints for twenty hours per day over several days. She was accompanied and supervised by staff every moment.

Years later, she was interviewed for an article in *Scientific American*. Legal scholar Elyn Saks is a law professor at the University of Southern California, a Marshall scholar, and a graduate of Yale Law School. In 2007, she published a frank and moving portrait of her experience with schizophrenia. *The Center Cannot Hold*[41] describes the outbreak of her illness in law school as a waking nightmare. In addition to delusions and hallucinations, her thinking was scrambled and illogical.

"My copies of the cases have been infiltrated. We have to case the joint. I don't believe in joints, but they do hold your body together."

---

[41] "Diary of a High-Functioning Person with Schizophrenia," Ellyn Saks; *Scientific American*, December 29, 2009.

She remembered the emotional distress, fear, and bodily pain of being physically restrained in the initial phase of her hospitalization. After several weeks, her symptoms went into remission. She was discharged. Subsequently, however, she did not do well until she finally accepted the need for therapy and medication.

"I stopped fighting the diagnosis and trying to prove by managing successfully without medication that I wasn't ill."

Following this insight, her life improved remarkably. She married, became a mother, and has pursued a fruitful career as an attorney and author. She has learned about her own illness in greater depth. She still has transient psychotic thoughts, sometimes several times a day, that she has killed people, but she is immediately aware that they are symptoms that can be dismissed. Three or four times yearly, she'll have periods of three or four days when psychotic thoughts become more pronounced in response to particular stresses, which she attempts to minimize by avoiding certain activities. Her law school has been flexible, permitting her to deemphasize classroom teaching and speaking engagements. Other aspects of her work—reading, researching, and writing—are gratifying.

She is able to reflect on schizophrenia as a researcher, interested author, and patient. She was fortunate she experienced largely positive and not negative symptoms, which can be more persistent and chronically disabling by eroding motivational drive and producing persistent apathy and incapacity to work or make friends. She has a message for so-called mental health professionals to immediately stop telling patients to drastically lower their expectations. With proper treatment and resources, people can reach their potential. She notes how devastated she was personally when she was told she was gravely ill and could not expect to support herself, marry, or live independently.

On a broader scale, she wants to educate the public that schizophrenia is not associated with violence; the predominant cause is substance abuse. Individuals with the illness basically are the same as everyone else: wishing not to suffer, seeking the fruits of a well-lived life, satisfying relationships, working, and finding pleasant leisure pursuits.

The professor was very fortunate. The illness struck when she had had the chance to plot her life path and rack up successes and accomplishments. The great majority of victims are cut down much earlier, often entering a period of sustained symptomatology and disability that they cannot overcome because of the gross inadequacies of the so-called mental health care system in accurately diagnosing the disease and efficiently starting comprehensive treatment. Many end up with the prognosis given to Professor Saks: a bleak and painful life. "I was also given a 'grave' prognosis. I was expected to be unable to live independently, let alone work."

No other disease strikes so savagely at the core of a human being, fragmenting the very capacity to know who one is in any positive or realistic sense. The disease bores a deep hole in which self-esteem and well-being no longer can reside. It turns the experience of life into a surrealistic desert in which sandstorms are whipped up unpredictably, obliterating sustaining emotions, love, positive beliefs, spirituality, and a sense of achievement and satisfaction. For these, it substitutes terror, persecution, failure, and isolation. To be in the grips of this disease is to be a participant in hell on this earth.

It is critical now—for the sake of hundreds of thousands to millions of those afflicted with schizophrenic-type illnesses—to finally decide if it is a mental health problem or a severe physical brain-based disorder. So many patients deteriorate, ending with crippled lives. If it is a mental problem, we can continue with the so-called mental health care system. If it's a severe brain disorder, it requires rapid diagnosis and competent treatment by a brain-oriented physicians. These brain psychiatrists have a deep specialist's knowledge of the brain mechanisms generating the symptoms and a wide understanding of how specific therapeutic approaches, predominantly with sophisticated pharmacology, but also psychosocial support, can prevent deterioration and promote well-being.

In the current mental health care system, rates of recovery in schizophrenia remain as low as 1–2 percent per year.[42] Tw- thirds of patients never marry, less than 15 percent hold competitive employment, and 20 percent are homeless at any point in time. The World Health Organization ranks schizophrenia as the third most disabling illness globally among adolescents through to middle age.

Much to the detriment of people with schizophrenia, who God knows are already racked with suffering from their so-called mental illness, the level of physical care they receive is far inferior to people in the physical care system. Dr. Michael H. Katz, deputy editor of *JAMA Internal Medicine* and director of the Los Angeles County Department of Health Services, said, "To improve care for persons with serious mental illness, it will be necessary to break down the silos that separate the mental health and physical health care systems."[43] Good luck with that. Who is keeping the silos separated? Organized psychiatry, which will never voluntarily relinquish its mental health bailiwick!

Since psychiatrists, by default, are the physicians who care for the physical health of their mental patients in their separate mental health care system, how are they doing? Their patients with schizophrenia have a twenty-five-year lower life expectancy than people in the general population.

In an original investigation[44] of 1,138,853 individuals with schizophrenia conducted in the United States from January 1, 2001, to December 31, 2007, it was determined people with schizophrenia were more than 3.5 times more likely to die during that period than people in the general population. Contrary to what people might think, suicide was the cause of death for a small minority, less than 5 percent. The great majority of deaths, 85 percent, were due to natural causes

[42] "Cognitive Impairment in Schizophrenia: Understanding the Neurobiology and Its Implications for Future Management." Supplement to *Current Psychiatry.* January 2015.

[43] "Clinical Psychiatry News Network." Shamon Aymes. *JAMA Internal Medicine.*

[44] "Premature Mortality among Adults with Schizophrenia in the United States," Olfson. M. et al. *JAMA Psychiatry.* Published online Oct. 28, 2015.

from cardiovascular disease, cancer, diabetes mellitus, hypertension, influenza, and pneumonia. In the remaining 15 percent of deaths due to unnatural causes, twice as many died from accidents compared to suicide. Drug and alcohol abuse-related deaths were also listed in the unnatural causes category.

The authors concluded excess cardiovascular mortality was evident even in young adults with schizophrenia. They concluded their findings highlight the importance of an early focus on primary prevention: the identification and management of conditions contributing to cardiovascular mortality risk, including diabetes mellitus, hypertension, hyperlipidemia, and other chronic diseases. Despite professional guidelines calling for screening of all psychiatric patients for tobacco use and providing evidence-based treatments for those interested in quitting, rates of screening and counseling for tobacco use and nicotine therapy remain low.[45]

The authors conclude because of the excess morbidity and mortality among individuals with schizophrenia, there must be earlier and more consistent management of their physical health.

The authors mean well, but they don't understand the mental health care system and psychiatrists. Theirs is a hollow exhortation to which most psychiatrists, particularly therapy psychiatrists, will pay little heed. Their great focus is their overriding mission to free their patients with schizophrenia from the deeply buried conflicts over aggression and sexuality.

There are 341 identified risk genes for the disease. Chromosome 6 has many of them. Compared to the general population, these genes increase the odds of developing schizophrenia by three to four times. In some instances, a mitosis abnormality also probably plays a role. Of the twenty thousand human genes, 50 percent, or half the total, code for the brain and its proteins, so 50 percent of all genetic mutations occur in genes coding for the brain. This can take the form of an abnormal number of alleles in genes: one or three versus the normal two copies.

---

[45] Ibid (3).

A number of external or environmental factors can play a role, influencing gene expression through epigenetic mechanisms: pregnancy complications, hypoxia during delivery, inadequate immunizations, poor prenatal care, vitamin D deficiency (incidence three times greater), paternal age greater than forty-five years (incidence three times greater), living in a large city (incidence four times greater), early life emotional traumas, abuse and stress, and childhood illnesses, including mood disorders. All these factors alter genes, resulting in abnormal cell development and programming and defective circuits in the brain, leading to symptomatic expression of the illness.

Modern neuroimaging technologies, functional MRI, MRS, and DTI, have permitted assessment of the brain in vivo. The technologies have progressed to the point that one cubic centimeter of brain tissue can be studied while an individual is engaged in different tasks and cognitive exercises, elucidating in more detail physical dysfunction in various brain areas. MRI permits assessment of blood flow and metabolic activity. DTI assesses white matter integrity. There are 137,000 kilometers of myelin fibers in the brain, sufficient to circle the earth three times! People with schizophrenia have a reduction in myelin by ten thousand kilometers—or more—and defects in its connectivity and structure. In addition, dendrites are deficient in the number of spines they form, thus diminishing available connecting points between neurons.

There is a multiplicity of additional abnormalities: reduction in neuroplasticity, increased apoptosis, decreased neurogenesis (partially attributable to decreased baby stem cell production in the dentate gyrus, hypothalamus, and subventricular zone). Baby stem cells are destined to produce mature neurons (50 percent of them) and glial cells (the other 50 percent). There are disturbances of metabolic functions: increased oxidative stress, excess production of free radicals, insufficient production of glutathione in mitochondria, decreased physical support of neurons in their local geography, and insufficient nutritional supplies, which all negatively affect neurons and glial cells. There are reductions in neurotropic factors—BDNF levels are 60 percent lower than normal—and the neurons have markedly reduced resistance to infection.

During psychotic episodes, there is an acceleration of the pathologies, and massive losses due to apoptosis accelerate the loss of brain tissue. Up to 5 percent by volume can be destroyed in each psychotic episode if effective treatment is not rapidly applied. One of the great tragedies of the current mental health care system is its gross deficiencies in diagnostic proficiency and the provision of timely suitable treatment. Most patients aren't seen until the disease has already progressed, much neuronal loss has occurred, and a lot of brain damage has been suffered. The deterioration is not generally reversible.

Community-functioning deficits in schizophrenia are apparent up to fifteen years before the first hospitalization. A study[46] was conducted in Israel of 723,316 Israeli male adolescents in which they were followed from the time they first visited their draft board for a mandatory behavioral health assessment and then for twenty-four years. Of that group, 3,929 individuals were hospitalized with schizophrenia. Impairments in social activity, independent behavior, and functioning at school or work were recognizable up to fifteen years before hospitalization.

If someone threatened to remove 5 percent of your brain, and then down the road escalated the threat to 10 percent, or 15 percent or more, there could be no greater nightmare, yet Dr. Nasrallah has educated us that each psychotic episode does precisely that. A system like the mental health care system—laid back, sloppy, and inexpert—poses a grievous threat to a person with schizophrenia. The disease destroys one's personal identity and one's very sense of self, and that is exactly what psychiatry does. Hapless patients bounce from one mental health provider to the next social worker, counselor,

---

[46] "Developmental Trajectories of Impaired Community Functioning in Schizophrenia." Dr. Keithorst, Eva Et al., *JAMA Psychiatry Online*, November 25, 2015.

psychologist, or therapy psychiatrist. There is no readily identifiable and available expert in the community such as the brain psychiatrist physician, who has a deep understanding of brain pathology and the differentiating, fine-tuned pharmacological treatments. Yes, the disease must be accurately diagnosed early on when it appears, the threat of brain damage acknowledged, and brain-specific treatments applied competently to prevent and resist it.

It requires an expert psychiatrist-physician (a brain psychiatrist) to pick up and diagnose the earliest manifestations of the disease—when there is still minimal brain damage. In the current mental health care system, there is usually a delay of several years after the onset of the earliest symptoms, *prodromal symptoms*, a cruel delay during which destructive brain processes are surging ahead without any competent attention.

The prodromal phase can be viewed as a sequence of subtly evolving symptoms,[47] termed *attenuated*, which the average so-called mental health provider may not recognize, view as significant, or comprehend as symptoms of an early schizophrenic illness. The positive attenuated symptoms include the appearance of unusual thoughts, emerging suspiciousness, perceptual abnormalities, and loosening of conceptual organization. The negative attenuated symptoms include initial withdrawal from social activities, a flattening of emotional expressiveness, depressed mood, and hints of deterioration in functioning. In the current mental health care system, this symptomatic phase can persist for years until the appearance of overt symptoms that are obvious to everyone. These psychotic symptoms result in crises and lead to an emergency situation that requires forceful involuntary hospitalization.

After the first psychotic episode, a further tragic tale of delay and treatment inadequacies propels the hapless patients—and their families—along a road with repeated stumbling, recurrent psychotic episodes, diminution in brain volume, and massive storms of apoptosis,

---

[47] "Schizophrenia Prodrome: An Optimal Approach," Madaan, V., MD, *Current Psychiatry,* March 13, 2014 (3)16–20, 20–30.

resulting in the destroyed end product: a totally devastated, disabled, miserable human being. Much of the essence of being human has been pulverized. It is not just their emotional, intellectual, and spiritual health; it is also their physical health.

Any young adult who is having these prodromal symptoms and the beginning of difficulties in academic and occupational functioning, or social withdrawal, who is in apparent distress, anxious or agitated, requires an expert brain psychiatrist to elicit and evaluate these early symptoms. They are a possible harbinger of a severe brain disorder, and brain tissue will be at risk unless appropriate treatment is prescribed. The brain psychiatrist must be clinically nimble enough to select and prescribe appropriate medications using lowest possible doses to control symptoms.

And the prescribing is delicate. Since there is a delayed therapeutic effect of up to several weeks, the prescriber must understand the pharmacodynamics and pharmacokinetics of medications to avoid overloading the medication, causing side effects, alienating the patient, and sentencing the patient to a lifetime of symptoms and suffering. The prescriber must take the time to educate the patient in the concepts of compliance and adherence to the medication schedule and explain why it is so critically important.

Research has shown that even relatively short gaps in treatment result in increased rates of psychotic episodes and hospitalizations. In one study,[48] 4,325 patients with schizophrenia were followed for a year (a relatively short period given the duration of the disease). In that period, compared to patients who took medication as prescribed, those who omitted medications from one to ten days had nearly double the number of hospitalizations during the year. For larger gaps of eleven to thirty days, it was nearly triple, and for gaps of greater than thirty days, hospitalizations were nearly quadruple.

The prescriber must understand how to track adherence, understanding that the failure of patients to reliably obtain and

[48] "Adherence, Recovery, and the Role of Loss in schizophrenia." Global Academy of Medical Education. September 18, 2014.

take medications as prescribed is a widespread issue in all medical specialties from cardiology to pulmonology. The characterization of so-called mental illness as mental—by psychiatrists—adds another formidable obstacle to promoting compliance. If these illnesses aren't even physical, why would medication even be necessary?

Tracking compliance requires medical expertise—the knowledge base of a brain psychiatrist who understands the importance of obtaining laboratory measurement of the concentrations in the blood of prescribed medication to assess compliance with the prescription and side effects to determine if blood levels are therapeutic but not toxic. It is critical to educate patients of the rationale for pharmacological decisions. Brain psychiatrists' knowledge of the specific brain mechanisms medications are intended beneficially to regulate will give evidence to the patient the prescriber is utilizing thought-out guidelines rather than mysterious guesswork.

The long-range management and treatment of schizophrenia in the current so-called mental health care system is even more catastrophic. For those patients fortunate enough to have a treatment-induced remission of their first psychotic episode, such success, as a rule, is soon followed by the discontinuation of antipsychotic medication, multiple relapses, progressive and refractoriness to treatment. The end stage of the disease is wreckage, a shell housing a decimated human being. Where once there were unique human characteristics, now there is a gray, drab, empty space filled with fear, depression, and terror.

Approximately 80 percent of patients relapse—half in less than two years. Each relapse exacerbates apoptosis, destroying up to 5 percent of the patient's brain tissue and yanking the victim out of all constructive, ego-rewarding pursuits, academics, work, relationships, and leisure interests, leaving a gaping void in their life trajectories. As this occurs, the so-called mental health care system is idling—unfocused and scattershot—as the affected individual wanders to therapists, counselors, emergency rooms, alternative approaches, and therapy psychiatrists.

What is required is a readily identifiable medical expert to whom patients and families can turn quickly. The brain psychiatrist understands the specific dysfunctional brain mechanisms that cause the symptoms and the complex pharmacology to stabilize them. The qualified brain psychiatrist can provide expert medical diagnosis and treatment in the same fashion as neurologists. After making a definitive and differential diagnosis, neurologists often refer to nonmedical providers, such as physical therapists. The brain psychiatrist would likewise refer for specialized psychotherapies by qualified social workers, counselors, and psychologists.

A medical treatment is available that only requires the patient to take medication very infrequently, even only quarterly, potentially greatly reducing noncompliance, relapses, and hospitalizations. Such specially formulated, long-acting medications must be given intramuscularly. Since they have a long duration of action, the side effects may also be stretched out. A high level of expertise is required of the prescriber, and this should always fall into the domain of the brain psychiatrist. In particular, many of the side effects are neurological. The brain psychiatrist, as part of their job description, must always have training in neurology.

Henry A. Nasrallah, MD, is the Sydney W. Sovers Professor and Chair in the Department of Neurology and Psychiatry at Saint Louis University School of Medicine. He is a graduate of a neuroscience fellowship at the National Institutes of Health, editor in chief of *Schizophrenia Research*, and cofounder of the Schizophrenia International Research Society. He has authored more than 360 scientific articles and eleven books. His research focus is the neurobiology and pharmacological treatment of schizophrenia. Dr. Nasrallah is informed about the real nature, symptoms, and causes of schizophrenia and does not consider schizophrenia a mental problem.

Clinically, it is an illness with many neurological symptoms. Individuals with schizophrenia have a number of neurological lesions.[49] Among them are neurological “soft signs,” which are any

---

[49] primeinc.org/62WB15/s

number of physical findings that collectively indicate the presence of neurological damage in the brain. These lesions are widely distributed in the brain rather than being localized. White matter containing the connecting cables between groups of neurons in different parts of the brain have physical damage and disruptions in its pathways. There are subtle abnormalities in the hippocampus and frontal lobes. There are subtle symptoms of neurological illnesses, particularly extrapyramidal symptoms and Parkinson's disease.

Prefrontal Cortex

Approximately 98 percent of patients have disturbances in cognitive capacity.[50] Cognition is defined as the ability to plan, attend to stimuli, filter out irrelevant stimuli, remember new information, engage in social interactions, and perform many other higher-order thought processes,[51] which make it possible to maintain adoptive functioning. Neuropsychological testing and other neurological parameters demonstrate how cognitive abnormalities are pervasive in schizophrenia and directly relate to impaired functioning.

Cognitive deficits are associated with dysfunction in many brain circuits in important brain regions, including the frontal cortex, hippocampus, and the auditory and parietal cortices. Neuroimaging studies and postmortem analyses demonstrate a reduction in whole brain volume, gray matter, and white matter. These analyses also reveal altered, disrupted synaptic connectivity involving the dopaminergic, glutamatergic, gamma amino butyric, and acetylcholinergic systems.

The neurotransmitter dopamine is elevated in the cortical and striatal regions. Two specific dopaminergic receptors—presynaptic and striatal D_0 receptors—are increased in number. The D-1 receptor, critical in maintaining normal dopaminergic neurotransmission

---

[50] "Cognitive Impairment in Schizophrenia: Understanding the Neurobiology and Its Implication for Future Management, Supplement, and Acelylcholinergic Systems."

[51] *Current Psychiatry*, Jan. 2015, 3. ibid, 2.

particularly in the prefrontal cortex (so important in cognitive functioning), does not function adequately. The approved pharmacological treatment of schizophrenia is with neuroleptic (antipsychotic) medication, which by blocking the D-2 receptor, reduces positive symptoms, but it has no direct benefit on cognitive or negative symptoms.

Neuroscientific research is making great progress with the eventual objective of reregulating nondopaminergic neurotransmission. Postmortem studies have demonstrated decreases of an important acetylcholinergic receptor, the a7, in the frontal cortex, striatum, and hippocampus in patients with schizophrenia. The a7 receptor seems particularly important for cognitive processing. Stimulating it results in overall enhancement of or improved regulation of GABAergic, glutaminergic neurotransmission in the hippocampus and midbrain, and improved synaptic connectivity. The end result can be improvements of memory functioning, emotional processing, enhanced motivational drive, and improved cognitive processing. Clinical trials are being conducted to develop new medications to target the a7 receptor, potentially opening up a new avenue to treat schizophrenia. High levels of expertise will be critical to understanding and utilizing these promising new medications.

GLOSSARY

dopamine. In the absence of sufficient serotonergic neurotransmission or its imbalance, dopamine becomes dominant.

neurobiological dysfunctions. Contribute to neuropsychological dysfunctions.

serotonin receptors. Proper balance between hippocampal 5-HT1A receptors and cortical 5-HT2A receptors is required for effective modulation of the stress reaction and inhibition of impulsivity and aggression (including suicidality).

serotonin 5-HT1A receptor. An important serotonin receptor playing a role in MDD and suicidality.

serotonin 5-HT2A receptor. Another important serotonin receptor playing a role in MDD and suicidality.

suicidality. Brain structures contributing to: right frontal lobes in association with the amygdalae, other limbic structures, the temporal lobes, and the hippocampus.

CHAPTER 17

Suicide

Life, to be alive, is a gift or should be considered as such. So why should any individual who chooses to depart from life be given any sympathy? An individual, by choosing this option, has revealed—for all to see—their cowardice, lack of fortitude, deficient will, and shabbiness of character. It seems logical that suicide is a manifestation of a mentally ill individual's very disturbed mind, and it is a feature of mental illness as opposed to physical illness.

Yes, there is a lot of harsh judgment directed at mentally ill individuals who attempt or complete suicide. Other individuals sick with physical illnesses such as diabetes, heart disease, cancer, or neurological diseases like multiple sclerosis, stroke, or epilepsy suffer far more than the mentally ill, but they bear up to their illnesses, never contemplating the coward's solution, even though they have real physical pain.

Do you mean individuals with real physical illnesses also may be suicidal? Nah! Oh, you say you'll force me to have an open mind by giving me the facts. I'm waiting.

Suicide risk is doubled in people with diabetes and cancer, and it's five times greater than in the general population for neurological disorders such as multiple sclerosis, spinal cord lesions, and stroke, and twenty-five times greater for difficult-to-treat epilepsy. No one would quibble that these are physical diseases of the body and brain.

Therapy psychiatrists believe the key to preventing suicide is the direct study of human emotions and deep conflicts in the unconscious. Children as young as three years old, however, can have suicidal thoughts. Have they had time to develop abnormal emotions and deep unconscious conflicts? It can't be denied that supportive therapy and helpful guidance is beneficial for suicidal individuals or that qualified psychologists and social workers can administer these. However, it should be common sense that an expert medical provider—a brain psychiatrist who understands the physical brain mechanisms predisposing individuals to become suicidal—should be readily identifiable and available, just as in neurology.

There is research evidence that individuals with major depression who are seriously suicidal have both neurobiological and neuropsychological differences from clinically depressed individuals who are not suicidal. Animal studies show that the proper balance between hippocampal 5-HT1A receptors and cortical 5-HT2A receptors is essential for adoptive neurobiological and neuropsychological modulation of the stress reaction and inhibition of impulsivity and aggression. Well-modulated serotonergic neurotransmission acts in an antagonistic way to dopamine so that if serotonin is depleted, relative dominance of dopamine occurs. When there is decreased binding to cortical, prefrontal 5-HT2 receptors, the serotonergic-dopaminergic balance is disturbed. Suicidal individuals may be more prone to incur this dysregulation.

The right front lobes in association with the amygdala, other limbic structures, the temporal cortices, and the hippocampus contribute to the vulnerability to suicidal behavior. The neurological dysfunctions are associated with neuropsychological (cognitive) ones.

Suicidal individuals have significant differences in some, though not all, neuropsychological tests. There are also three cognitive characteristics that are more pronounced. The first is an extreme hypersensitivity to rejection and criticism in interpersonal and social contexts. The second is an extreme block to problem-solving thinking, the inability to think out solutions, and the inability to think of rescue factors that might occur in the future.

Attention is heavily directed at painful or distressing events. Memory is selective for the most disturbing past events. Fluency, the ability to turn one's thinking around to conceptualize positive outcomes, is disabled. The cumulative result is profound hopelessness.

For those who have contempt for individuals who would stoop to suicide, it might be enlightening to consider suicidality among veterans, particularly the ones who have served in active combat, having placed their lives, limbs, security, and comfort in such danger. Through their exploits in combat, haven't they proven they are not lacking in courage, grit, and intelligence? Well, the first grisly act against these soldiers is to call them mentally ill to begin with. Psychiatry, by asserting its favorite label, undoubtedly scares away thousands of soldiers who can't accept they are mental. What combat veteran wants to associate himself with people they believe are crazy people, ne'er-do-wells, goof-offs, and gutless? It is best to avoid the stinking mental health care system entirely if at all possible. Many, of course, will pay a very heavy price for avoiding the stigma, thereby never receiving treatment.

Marine Clay Hunt received a hero's welcome when he returned home from Afghanistan where he served as a sniper.[52] He had received a purple heart. He had been diagnosed with PTSD, but heaven only knows how competent his mental health care providers were, particularly after he left the service. After his honorable discharge, he was widely recognized as an advocate for veterans. However, two years after his discharge, the twenty-eight-year-old committed suicide, one of the eight thousand veterans who commit suicide each year.

Preventing military suicides is described as a national health concern and a health priority.[53] From January 1, 2004, through

---

[52] "22 Veterans Commit Suicide Each Day." Justin Worland@justinworland, Feb. 6, 2015.

[53] "Suicide Attempts in the US Army During the Wars in Afghanistan and Iraq, 2004–2009." Ursano, B. J. et al. *JAMA Psychiatry*, July 8, 2015.

December 31, 2009, the army experienced a sustained increase in nonfatal and fatal suicides among soldiers who had been in combat, particularly among enlisted soldiers. The researchers who investigated this concluded it is critical for providers (whoever they are!) to accurately determine those who are at greatest risk, employing enhanced surveillance and evidence-based prevention targeting. Fat chance that will work! As long as soldiers are forced to swallow that seeking treatment will pigeonhole them as mental cases, courtesy of psychiatry, the loss of veterans through suicide will grind on. Also, who knows what type of mental health provider they'll encounter.

Extreme hopelessness is the handmaiden of suicide.

The Black Pit

In severe major depression, the accompaniment of neurobiological dysregulation can result in a sort of brain freeze. Certain cognitions (severe negative neuropsychological cognitive content) becomes as if set in concrete, taking on an extreme intensity and a fixity, rising like a gusher from the emotional brain (the limbic system) to flood logical reasoning (largely a cortical function).

Encouraging an individual in the grips of such tenacious cognitions and their belief content, to simply get on with it, is as logical as informing the water bursting forth from a dam to recede. Such advice, even well-intentioned advice, is like criticizing an individual caught in the flow of rampaging water to just get over it. The cognitions are of an extreme catastrophic nature. Everything of value—their own positive identity, relationships, occupational status, and health—are being decimated. That they will end up helpless, totally disabled, in a barren state hospital room or dead to the outsider can appear ridiculous, but in the cognitive black pit, it is a reality for the sufferer. The black pit cognitive phenomenon is accompanied by equivalently catastrophic emotions of fear, horror, dread, and profound hopelessness. That is what occurs in severe major depression.

CHAPTER 18

Violence

Aren't many mental patients violent? You see it all the time on TV—all those vicious serial murderers. They're all mentally ill.

The *Wall Street Journal* ran an editorial, Mass Murder Returns: Another Case of Mental Illness and Violence, on April 4, 2014:

> The shooting and deaths Wednesday at Fort Hood, Texas, return an array of grim memories and tough questions to public attention. This is the same place where Army Major Nidal Massan massacred soldiers and civilians in 2009. That was a terrorist attack for which Hassan was convicted of murder last August ... more protection from severe and out of control mental illness.
>
> The protection should include laws requiring extremely ill patients to receive assisted outpatient treatment. Those who refuse need to be committed to a hospital for care. The most troubled, anxious, and depressed individuals to often don't get the focused attention and counseling needed to break their fall. We lives in a time when attention is paid to and public money spent on all manner of personal grievance and

> injury—severe mental illness is not one of them. It should be.
>
> Whether the extent into extreme violence occurs on a military base or at a civilian workplace, school or shopping center is a subordinate concern to the reality of mentally ill individuals going on killing sprees. We do know about the (11) other killers, in Newtown, Aurora, Tucson and Virginia Tech. to know society deserves …

Is mental illness the guilty culprit in mass shootings and gun violence in general? The psychiatrists have nothing to say on the issue. The mentally ill may or may not be savage slaughterers, but organized psychiatry is peepless. God forbid they should sponsor a mass education campaign to educate the public. What is it to them if the mentally ill, if they are not actually murdering brutes in reality, are burdened even more with stigma, humiliation, suspicion, and rejections if the public thinks of them as such?

In the ***Wall Street Journal***'s article, "A Proposal to Reduce Gun Violence by the Mentally Ill," the author presents an outline for a program to reduce gun violence by the mentally ill, assuming the assertion by the *WSJ* editorial page that gun violence is attributable to the mentally ill is accurate. The program would proceed in stages:

1. Create a federal registry of all the individuals currently receiving mental health treatment by mandating all therapists and mental health providers submit the names of their clients/patients and relevant associated clinical information directly to the registry for incorporation into its unified database.
2. Since a significant proportion of mentally ill individuals have never entered treatment, a method of mass screening of the entire population will be devised employing online and/or written screening examinations (the latter being mailed, employing the latest census data) to all individuals over ten

years of age who have not submitted an online screening examination. If the screening material indicates the presence of mental illness, the names and relevant clinical information of such individuals will also be incorporated into the federal registry.

3. All individuals entered into the federal registry will have restrictions governing their purchase of any weapon, will be required to surrender any weapons in their possession, and will have to submit to mental health evaluations to obtain clearance for the purchase of weapons.

Actually, it is not just the *WSJ* that attributes gun violence to the mentally ill. The media as a whole, particularly the visual media, like ravenous vultures, descend on high-profile mass shootings, obsessively and repetitively broadcasting images and news content, intimate details of the killer(s), the specifics of the weapons used, including information of how they were acquired and armed. In almost all such cases, the killer is portrayed as a mentally ill outcast.

Unfortunately, even some prominent individuals who bear no malice toward the mentally ill seem to believe that gun violence is linked to mental illness. When Representative Tim Murphy, PhD, first introduced the Helping Families in Mental Health Crises Act in December 2013, he opened his speech by mentioning the Sandy Hook Elementary School mass shooting catastrophe in Newton, Connecticut. "If we want to prevent Newtowns, Tucsons, Auroras, Pittsburghs, and Columbines, we have to do something comprehensive, research-based, and we have to do it now.[54] And when Senator Bill Cassidy, MD, and Senator Chris Murphy discussed the Mental Health Reform Act, they also raised the specter of mass shootings. According to Cassidy, a gastroenterologist, the act attempts to address the root cause of mass violence, which is recognized but untreated mental illness.[55]

---

[54] "Mental Health Reform Will Not Reduce U.S. Gun Violence, Experts Say." Rubin, Rita, MA. *JAMA* published online December 16, 2015.

[55] Ibid.

Actually, high-profile mass shootings represent a tiny fraction of gun-inflicted homicides, about 4 percent. Through early December 2015, a total of 450 individuals perished in mass shootings; the rest, 11,208, died in more ordinary gun-related killings.[56] Interestingly, a meta-analysis of studies from Europe determined the risk of an individual with schizophrenia killing a stranger in a given year is 1 in 70,000 patients.[57]

Scientists who study gun violence say whatever the benefits of mental health reform, it won't make much of a dent in the number of homicides and attempted homicides committed with firearms because of the vast majority of perpetrators are not mentally ill. The mentally ill are far more likely to be victims. An expert, psychiatrist Jonathan Metzl, MD, PhD, has noted there is no real psychiatric diagnosis that psychiatrists can use to predict which patient is going to become violent. By blaming gun violence on mental illness, we lose the sense of the larger contextual factors that surround violence,[58] such as drinking, arguments, having access to firearms, and having a history of violence, all of which are statistically correlated with gun violence but not linked to mental health disorders.

There may be far more evidence-based approaches to reducing gun violence than blaming mental illness. A definitive study, "Guns, Impulsive Angry Behavior, and Mental Disorders: Results from the National Comorbidity Survey Replication,"[59] was summarized in the Huffington Post on December 24, 2015: "Harvard Study Finds Anger Issues, Not Major Mental Illness, Tied to Gun Violence." Five thousand five hundred sixty-three face-to-face and household interviews and assessments were conducted. The respondents' mental health, patterns

---

[56] Ibid.

[57] Ibid.

[58] Ibid.

[59] Jeffrey W. Swanson, Jeffrey W. et al [Nancy A. Sampson, Maria V. Petukhova, Alan M. Zestavsky, Paul S. Appelbaum, Marvin S. Swartz, Ronald C. Kessler]. "Guns, Impulsive Angry Behavior, and Mental Disorders: Results from the National Comorbidity Survey Replication" (NCS-R). *Behavioral Sciences and the Law*, 2015; DO1: 10, 1002/bal. 2172

of impulsive anger, how many guns they owned, and whether they carried guns outside of the home were determined. One of the most significant findings was the correlation of gun violence with three attributes of individuals at greater risk of gun violence. The first was ownership of multiple guns, the second was carrying a gun outside of the home, and finally was a pattern of angry, impulsive behavior. Study participants who owned six or more guns were four times more likely to carry guns outside the home and be in the high-risk anger group. The study found little overlap between having a major mental illness like schizophrenia or bipolar disorder and being impulsive, anger-prone, and having access to firearms. This comprehensive study corroborated previous research indicating the great majority of people with mental illness is not likely to be violent since only 4 percent of such violence is attributable to major mental illness.[60]

Jeffrey Swanson, PhD, professor of psychiatry and behavioral sciences at Duke University School of Medicine and lead author of the Harvard study has observed that we tend to focus on the issue of gun violence only after a horrifying mass casualty shooting in which any sense of proportion is completely lost in the shuffle. "Mental illness and gun violence are two very complicated population health problems that come together only on their edges."[61] If there are a tiny minority of people with mental illness, weapons, and serious anger problems, blaming mental illness for gun violence only increases the stigma and reinforces avoidance of evaluation and treatment.

An important conclusion of the study authors is that a more effective policy measure would be to restrict gun access based on an individual's arrest history. Arrests could indicate a history of impulsive or angry behavior, for example, criminal records of misdemeanor violence, DWIs, domestic violence, and restraining orders would serve as more relevant indications of gun violence risk. Swanson summarized the group we should focus on has impulsive or angry

---

[60] *Huffington Post*, December 24, 2015. "Harvard Study Finds Anger Issues, Not Major Mental Illness, Tied to Gun Violence."

[61] Ibid (Harvard).

behavior far beyond regular angry behavior: "The most volatile people are slipping through the cracks."[62]

The Accomplice

In *Forbes*, Joseph Granny wrote "The Media Is an Accomplice in Public Shootings: A Call for the 'Stephen King Law.'" It examined the losses and suffering of the victims and their families and the horror of witnessing the media broadly publicizing the grisly details. For example, naming the shooter, giving details of his personal characteristics—age, ethnicity, race—his gun-purchasing history, the details of the crime, the body count, and comparisons to previous perpetrators, including rankings of successful attackers. After every mass shooting, he hopes and prays the media won't amplify the violence, but they always proceed to do so. The effect of mass publicity on causing spikes in both celebrity suicides and mass violence has been understood for nearly forty years. For example, a well-known suicide serves as a model for additional suicides.[63] In the month after Marilyn Monroe's suicide, researchers noted an increase of two hundred suicides.

Mass shootings are better seen not as isolated events but acts built upon blueprints of previous rampages.[64] Christopher Harper-Mercer, the perpetrator of a mass shooting at an Oregon community college in September 2015, had uploaded a video about the 2012 massacre at Sandy Hook Elementary School in Newtown, Connecticut. The perpetrator of that massacre had studied the 1999 shootings at Columbine High School in Colorado in which thirteen people died, and the slaughter in 2011 in which seventy-seven people were killed.

Dr. Deborah Weisbrot, an associate clinical professor of psychiatry at Stony Brook University has interviewed hundreds of mostly teenage

---

[62] Ibid (Harvard).

[63] Copycat suicide, Wikipedia, December 26, 2015.

[64] "Mass Killings Are Seen as a Kind of Contagion." Goode, E. and Cadrey, Benedict. *The New York Times*, October 7, 2015.

boys after they made serious threats. "If you blast the names and faces of shooters on news stations and constantly repeat their names, there may be an inadvertent process of creating a blueprint."[65]

Dr. Robert A. Fein, a psychologist whose specialty is target violence, said, "You'd have a hard time finding someone who didn't do research about those who went before."

Dr. Keith Cameron, director of the Canadian Center for Threat Assessment, said, "The more they identify with the characteristics of the story, the more it will increase their level of risk."[66]

Peter Blair, director of the Advanced Law Enforcement Rapid Response Training Center at Texas State University started a campaign called Don't Name Them,[67] a policy in which Sheriff John Hanlin of Douglas County, Oregon, asked the news media to follow in the Oregon case—with little success.

Several localities have adopted broad and coordinated prevention measures. In Los Angeles County, a triad of law enforcement officials, educational institutions, and the county mental health department officials have coordinated efforts to share information and train staff members to recognize and report worrisome behavior. (This author notes that leaving the matter solely under the auspices of mental health is plainly stupid and dangerous!) In the weeks immediately after a mass shooting, they act proactively and closely monitor young people who could be at risk to act out as copycats. Dr. Beliz, identified in the *Times* article, is quoted as saying there have been no mass shootings in places where the Los Angeles program has been in operation.

Mr. Grenny concludes that although the media appropriately defends its right to fully participate in the marketplace of ideas,[68] in the matter of speech that leads to verifiable harm, it is time to discuss limits. When speech incites crime or influences harm, there must

---

65 Ibid.

66 Ibid.

67 Ibid.

68 "The Media Is an Accomplice in Public Shootings: A Call for a 'Stephen King Law.'" Grenny, Joseph, December 13, 2012, www.forbes.com/sites/josephgrenny/)

be limitations on it. Media moguls have had thirty-eight years to consider the ethical implications of their behavior in the matter of mass shootings, and they have been found wanting in accepting their responsibility. He said, "We need to discuss the merits and morality of appropriate legislation in the matter."

GLOSSARY

axon fibers, myelinated. The axon is a long, slender projection from the nerve cell that is protected by a myelin sheath, a fatty substance that serves as an electrically insulating layer.

deafferentation. A loss of sensory input caused by injury of nerves from the body.

executive function. A set of cognitive processes allowing attentional control, inhibitory control, working memory, reasoning, problem-solving, and planning.

frontal, parietal, temporal regions. Three of the major lobes of the cortex.

histopathological changes. Abnormalities in body tissues when viewed through a microscope (at the cellular level).

medial prefrontal cortex. An important part of the frontal cortex that mediates decision-making.

myelin synthesis. Two types of cells, Schwann cells and oligodendrocytes, supply the myelin for the axons.

orbital frontal cortex. A prefrontal cortex region involved in cognitive processing and decision-making.

sleep. Deep stages (non-REM slow-wave) sleep. The deepest, most restful level of sleep. It can be detected with the EEG (electroencephalogram).

poor sleep quality. Insomnia, interrupted sleep. There is generally a deficiency in slow-wave sleep. There can be serious consequences, increased risk for disease, accidents, and impaired performance. With increasing age, apoptosis.

synaptic density. A protein-based specialization of the synapse, enhancing synaptic transmission.

CHAPTER 19

Sleep

Claire E. Sexton, et al, studied the relationship between sleep quality and cortical and hippocampal volume.[69] Previous research had linked difficulties in initiating or maintaining sleep (nonrestorative sleep) to cognitive decline and deficits and Alzheimer's disease. Even primary insomnia (insomnia that is not accompanied by psychiatric or neurodegenerative diseases) had been linked to reductions of brain volume in important brain regions, the orbital frontal cortex, hippocampus, and precuneus. Reductions in non-REM slow-wave activity (the deep stages of sleep) had been linked in older adults with greater than normal age-related reductions in brain matter density (decreases in neurons) in the medial prefrontal cortex.

Dr. Sexton's group studied 147 adults living in their communities over three and a half years. They utilized an instrument to measure the quality of sleep, the Pittsburgh Sleep Quality Index, which measures domains of sleep quality (duration, subjective sleep quality, latency, habitual sleep efficiency, sleep disturbances, use of sleeping medication, and daytime dysfunction).

They measured brain volume with MRI scans at the initiation of and the end of the study, measuring both cross-sectional and longitudinal volumes. The results were very significant for those sixty

[69] Sexton, Claire E, reference, et al. "Poor sleep quality is associated with increased cortical atrophy in community-dwelling adults."

or older. Poor sleep quality was correlated with more atrophy within the orbital frontal cortex and the frontal, parietal, and temporal regions of the brain. These structural changes have been linked to decreases in cognitive performance, impairment of executive functions, and visual-spatial reasoning abilities across the life span.

Histopathological changes in brain tissue included shrinkage of large neurons, loss of myelinated axon fibers, and deafferentation and reductions in synaptic density. The authors comment that sleep has been proposed to be the brain's housekeeper, serving to restore and repair the brain, and enhancing the removal of potentially neurotoxic waste products, and an increase in the expression of genes related to myelin syntheses and maintenance. It follows that poor sleep may have a direct impact on brain structure.[70] They do note this pathological process may consist of a destructive feedback loop; as brain structure is negatively impacted, this further impairs sleep quality. They state the relationship between sleep quality and brain atrophy is not influenced by physical activity levels, weight, or blood pressure, and they particularly note the relationship between poor sleep quality and brain atrophy as a prominent issue in both psychiatric and neurodegenerative diseases.

Oh, so what's a shrunken brain? It's only a mental problem. Pull yourself together and snap out of it!

Is poor sleep a mental problem in which lurking unconscious conflicts arise during the night and awaken the victim? Well, that's what psychiatry thinks. At least they no longer believe that stirring demons are the cause of insomnia.

Unfortunately, insomnia is a core symptom of most major so-called mental disorders. In severe cases, it doubles the misery of the active illness. Severe panic attacks can abruptly occur during sleep, startling a person awake. These are nocturnal panic attacks. The individual experiences a surge of intense fear, which transitions to a state of terror in a matter of seconds: pounding heart, cold sweats, dizziness, chest pain, nausea, and numbness. Most frightening is the

---

[70] Ibid.

feeling of smothering and the certain belief of impending death. These symptoms are amazingly similar to the effects of waterboarding.

Christopher Hitchens, the deceased author and celebrity, voluntarily subjected himself to waterboarding. He was given a metal object to drop when the distress became overwhelming. Individuals skilled in administering the procedure placed the towel over his face and proceeded to pour water over it. Hitchens dropped the metal object after fifteen seconds, and the cloth was pulled from his face. "Well, then, if waterboarding does not constitute torture, then there is no such thing as torture."[71]

Panic attacks can occur in the context of any mental disorder, anxiety disorders, depressive disorders, bipolar disorders, eating disorders, and psychotic disorders. They can occur nocturnally, ravaging the sleep of the sufferers. It is impossible to settle down into a peaceful, restful restorative sleep afterward, and sufferers can become phobic about falling asleep.

Insomnia, even when not provoked by nocturnal panic attacks, can feel like a degree of torture. Anticipation of not sleeping can produce an inner pressure to get to sleep, which paradoxically produces an excitatory state in the body, which militates against getting to sleep. As frustration and desperation build, the individual becomes more restless, impatient, and frustrated. If the individual finally gets to sleep, the sleep feels short-circuited, superficial, and restless. There is an inability to get down to a deeper, more restful stage of sleep. The individual would give anything to fall into a deeper sleep. There are also many awakenings throughout the very long, unpleasant night. The following day brings fatigue, lack of energy, drowsiness, loss of enthusiasm and enjoyment, body aches and pains, general dysphoria, and an absent sense of well-being.

Psychiatry insists insomnia is really just a mental problem. Is the health and integrity of the physical brain caught up in the misery of insomnia? Is insomnia a symptomatic issue associated with physical brain dysfunction?

---

[71] Waterboarding. From Wikipedia, the free encyclopedia.

GLOSSARY

amyloid-beta peptides. Composed of thirty-six to forty-three amino acids involved in Alzheimer's disease by forming destructive amyloid plaques and impairing neuron structure and function.

amyloid precursor protein. A protein from which amyloid-beta peptides are constructed.

hyperphosphorylation of tau. It forms microtubules that give shape to neurons. In the process of hyperphosphorylation, excess tau forms neurofibrillary tangles that strangle neurons.

N-acetyl aspartate. An amino acid derivative associated with the health of neurons.

neurofibrillary tangles. Aggregates of hyperphosphorylated tau protein, which is a primary marker for Alzheimer's disease.

CHAPTER 20

Expertise

Making an accurate diagnosis is the keystone of medical practice because there follows from it the highest likelihood of recommending treatments that will have the highest probability of success. In general medicine, the well-trained practitioner never decides on a particular diagnosis without reviewing a list of diagnoses that could conceivably account for a patient's symptoms. That weighing is termed *making a differential diagnosis*. This is very important because different diseases can mimic one another but require different treatment approaches.

It is very difficult for a layperson or patient to assess a physician's accuracy in the diagnostic process; it is basically a matter of trust. Fortunately, in general medicine, the steps of diagnosis and differential diagnosis are drilled into physicians in internship and residency training programs, and they are expected to rigorously adhere to a disciplined approach that will guide them in ordering relevant laboratory examinations.

Unfortunately, psychiatry—isolated in its own mental health care system—has a much less rigorous approach. This is especially true for therapy psychiatrists, particularly those who are older and more distant from training. Psychiatry training programs (residencies), although there is some recent improvement in quality, overall emphasize psychoanalytic conceptualizations, which completely deemphasize the diagnostic process.

A mental patient with a serious disorder is exposed to decidedly nonmedical approaches to diagnosis since most lay therapists and therapy psychiatrists lack training and experience in such a vital matter. Such providers may not even utilize diagnostic concepts (except to guess at a diagnostic code for insurance purposes). They may just pick a common diagnosis without reviewing the diagnostic criteria or making a differential diagnosis. Its catch as catch can!

In modern neuroscience, accuracy of diagnosis is critical. The brain, as much or more than any other body part or organ, demands the same rigorous disciplined medical approach in the diagnostic evaluation and workup.

Actually, even in psychiatry, there are diagnostic tools available to assess and measure all possible symptoms and illnesses. The problem is that most psychiatrists do not use them! The average psychiatrist, during an initial evaluation, will just decide on a convenient diagnosis without working his way through a differential diagnosis. He will conduct a loose conversation with the patient, devoid of the disciplined questions that are essential for an accurate diagnostic process.

Actually, it is now possible for patients to make their own diagnosis and bring the results into the psychiatrist! (Although the psychiatrist may slough it off). Any serious psychiatrist actually should require patients to fill it out as part of an initial evaluation. The MINI-International Neuropsychiatric Interview is a structured diagnostic interview developed to assess the diagnoses of psychiatric patients. It can be used for research purposes, but because of its brevity—twenty to thirty minutes—it is especially convenient for diagnosing psychiatric patients in the practice setting. It is available online and can be printed out as a PDF. Actually, it is a sin if a psychiatrist does not utilize it!

A competent psychiatrist must also be a competent physician, putting particular emphasis on not isolating himself from the practice of medicine as so many therapy psychiatrists do. As should be obvious by now, human diseases do not arrange themselves according to the psychological needs of therapy psychiatrists by keeping a clear dividing line between mental and physical diseases. A multiplicity of physical diseases masquerade as mental problems.

Does the psychiatrist know? The psychiatrist sees the following patients in an initial evaluation:

A middle-aged man complains of boredom, insomnia, fatigue, and irritability. He is apparently depressed. Does the psychiatrist know that depression can be caused by a low calcium level? Will that cross his mind if the patient has an insufficient improvement on a trial of an antidepressant? Does he know how to rule out the causes of low calcium and which laboratory tests to order? (Serum calcium and phosphate and a parathyroid hormone level).

Another patient reports feeling very irritable. He appears suspicious and guarded. He feels ill at ease and is certain people are constantly looking at him in an accusatory fashion. If it is determined he is having borderline psychotic symptoms—but does not improve adequately on a low dosage of a second-generation antipsychotic—does the psychiatrist know this different set of symptoms can be caused by low calcium?

A middle-aged man complains of low energy, insomnia, decreased concentration, and low libido. Could borderline testosterone levels be implicated?

Another middle-aged man is diagnosed with depression, and he also has diabetes. Does the psychiatrist consider the cause of the diabetes in addition to depression? Does he know depression can seriously worsen diabetes? Will he be aware of the dangers of severe hypoglycemia?

Another middle-aged man complains of boredom, irritability, insomnia, and reduced libido. Should a testosterone level be considered? Does the psychiatrist obtain a blood pressure reading? Does he inquire about the presence of medical and neurological disease? Hypertension in the presence of depression significantly increases, nearly doubling, the probability of heart attack, stroke, heart failure, and cardiovascular death. Is the psychiatrist aware of this?

Seizures and Suicide

For the individual who has had a seizure, there is an effective, direct route to medically competent providers who are skilled in assessment and treatment. For practical patient care, it is considered of primary importance to diagnose specific seizure types and syndromes that inform etiology, treatment, and prognosis. From the beginning of the onset of the seizure disorder, the neurologist is consulted first. He immediately takes a history and performs a physical examination to establish a differential diagnosis and orders diagnostic and laboratory tests. Then, with medically relevant data at his disposal, he formulates a tailored plan for the prescription of pharmaceuticals.

A patient with latent suicidality, which he or she may not be fully conscious of, may not have the experience to assess or may not want to acknowledge. Suicide is the second-leading cause of death of fifteen-to-thirty-four-year-olds, claiming more than eleven thousand lives in that age group annually. For every completed suicide, there have been at least ten attempts. Those individuals do not have the equivalent of a neurologist to consult with expeditiously. Instead, there is a confusing array of providers. Should it be a counselor, a teacher, a family doctor, a social worker, a faith healer, a family member, a psychologist, or a therapy psychiatrist?

None of the above. It must be the neurologist equivalent: the brain psychiatrist. The expert is intimately knowledgeable about the relationship of symptoms of so-called mental illness to pathological brain mechanisms, who is skilled in differential diagnosis, and the pharmaceutical choices available to alleviate the acute symptoms of the illness diagnosed. In other words, the epileptic must consult with the neurologist before the physical therapist, nutritionist, occupational therapist, neuropsychologist, sleep specialist, pharmacist, radiologist, movement-disorder specialist, or the specialist who administers deep-brain stimulation.

Conducting an effective interview to assess suicidal risk requires a high degree of training and expertise; it is not a casual or informal process. Since suicidality is a symptom of several serious psychiatric disorders, it makes no sense if the clinician is not first and foremost an expert diagnostician who is able to accurately formulate a differential diagnosis, including active symptoms of psychiatric illness and medical, neurological, and endocrine illnesses, possibly precipitating the suicidality. That should be the brain psychiatrist.

Shawn Christopher Shea, MD, in an article in the *Psychiatric Times*,[72] focuses on the detailed set of interviewing skills needed to effectively elicit suicidal ideation, behaviors, and intent. It's the validity of the information acquired that is so important in determining as accurately as possible the risk of imminent suicide. He states as any supervisor will testify, "There is little doubt that two clinicians, after eliciting suicidal ideation from the same patient, can walk away with surprisingly different information."

This is true in the current mental health care system in which a smorgasbord of mental health providers, many with limited experience and training, perhaps limited to a bachelor's degree, conduct the initial interviews and evaluations.

Dr. Shea says a sound suicide assessment approach or protocol is made up of three components. The first is obtaining information about warning signs of suicide, risk factors, and protective factors. The second is collecting information about the patient's suicidal ideation, planning, behaviors, and level of intent. The final is making a clinical formulation to guide treatment decisions.

He points out many patients may withhold information for a variety of reasons. Some are determined to die and have completely given up hope of getting relief. They may not want to disclose their true intent and plans to prevent interference. Others may be ashamed of suicidal thoughts or think they're immoral, not a fitting topic for discussion, or synonymous with being crazy. They might anticipate the police will be notified—and they'll be locked up.

Therefore, it is critical to be aware the patient's stated intent may

---

[72] Shea, S. C., "Uncovering Suicidal Intent: A Sophisticated Art," *Psychiatric Times*: vol. 26, No. 12, December 3, 2009.

not reflect the actual intent, which the doctor terms *reflected intent*. Not to keep this in mind can result in a gross underestimation of the risk. He gives an example of a patient who did admit to having a plan to overdose, but after talking with the therapist, acknowledged feeling better. Several days later, however, his girlfriend ended their relationship. The patient shot himself. A psychological postmortem revealed he kept guns and had been observed handling one—and even loading it. His suicidal ideation had become acute after his girlfriend's rejection. He had not disclosed the second, more lethal means of suicide.

Reflected intent is the quality and quantity of the patient's suicidal thoughts, plans, and degree of action taken to complete the plans. The extent of the effort and time invested in making suicidal plans is a better measure of risk than the stated intent. Eliciting such reflections of intent through skillful interviewing may be lifesaving.

The clinician must also keep in mind the patient may have a miraculous cure and then unpredictably clam up, setting himself up for massive disillusionment. If at all possible, it is critical to estimate the credibility of the patient's self-report by seeking collaborative sources of information (spouse, family members, therapists). One study of completed suicides showed 60 percent of patients had communicated suicidal thoughts to a spouse and 50 percent to a relative.

A major decision the clinician must make is whether to hospitalize a patient, and the patient might be very unhappy. It is far easier and preferable if the patient cooperates, diminishing the tribulations of an involuntary hospitalization. Developing a degree of rapport and rationally framing the reasons for hospitalization in terms of the patient's self-interest are also served by a high level of expertise.

A simple molecule—a safe, inexpensive but efficacious one—is rarely prescribed by psychiatrists in the United States, only 7.5 percent utilizing it in treatment.[73] In England, the comparable utilization is 50 percent. In England, psychiatrists are inclined to identify with medicine rather than therapy. They evidently have less of a need to

[73] "Reappraisal." *British Journal of Psychiatry*, vol. 191, Issue 6, Aug. 22, 2007.

be semi-philosophers probing the depths of the human psyche, the practitioners of a highfalutin psychoanalytic therapy relieving their patients' sufferings by dispensing profound interpretations to suck out deeply buried unconscious conflicts in the id and superego.

Well, why don't psychiatrists prescribe lithium? Well, you have to be a real doctor, familiar with the organs of the body in addition to the brain, and able to order laboratory tests and interpret their results. That is just too grubby for most of them.

Lithium is an old drug that got a bad reputation. Psychiatrists in this country who prescribed it thirty or forty years ago were very clumsy in the prescription and monitoring of it. There were side effects—often serious ones. However, lithium can be prescribed safely if you're willing to be a physician and practice real medicine!

So why is lithium important? A meta-analysis of fourteen randomized, controlled trials provides strong evidence of its efficacy of preventing relapse to any mood episode in major mood illnesses, bipolar and/or unipolar. In particular, it cuts the incidence of suicide and suicidality by nearly 80 percent! Cipriani et al. (2005) and Baldessarini et al (2006) found lithium reduces the risk of suicide to an odds ratio of .26. That means for every hundred suicides before the prescription of lithium, there were only twenty-six after its prescription. This is quite obviously a tremendous sparing of risk for fatalities.

In addition, lithium also reduces the lethality of suicide attempts. The ratio of attempts to completed suicides for bipolar disorder is 5:1 in contrast to 20–30:1 for the general population. The prescription of lithium improves the ratio for bipolar disorder to 15–1, which is still not as favorable as the general population ratio is but significantly life-and-injury saving.

It is believed lithium has neuroprotective properties if knowledgably and safely prescribed and monitored. These neuroprotective effects include blocking accumulation of amyloid-beta peptides that overproduce amyloid precursor protein in the brains of people with Alzheimer's disease, inhibiting hyperphosphorylation of tau, the main component of neurofibrillary tangles, antagonizing vinca alkaloid neurotoxicity, which causes nerve and muscle damage, increasing N-acetyl-aspartate in all brain regions, a potential marker of neuronal viability and function, and increasing gray matter volume. Individuals with bipolar disorder have a significantly higher incidence of Alzheimer's disease in contrast to the general population. The prescription of lithium normalizes this greater risk.

In general medicine, competent physicians understand that many classes of drugs that treat serious diseases also carry risks of serious side effects. That does not mean they will not prescribe proven medications. They manage risk by weighing the risks and benefits of what they prescribe and then carefully monitoring the patient's status on such medications, evaluating symptoms and changes, employing questioning, history, physical examinations, and laboratory studies. Perhaps if they were practicing like psychiatrists; they just would not prescribe certain antibiotics, anti-inflammatory or anti-cancer drugs! (There can be serious adverse effects, and they would not bother to order laboratory tests).

The lifesaving drug lithium can have serious side effects. Yes, lithium must be prescribed and monitored carefully. When starting lithium, a complete battery of laboratory tests, standard for a physical examination, should be ordered. Lithium levels should be ordered until the lithium blood levels are in the range of 0.5 and 0.8 m Eq./L. Then expert clinical judgment will next determine when a further increase is indicated to .8–1 m Eq./L. There are comprehensive guidelines for the prevention, monitoring, and treatment of adverse effects. Therefore, there can be no excuse for any medical specialty not being trained and drilled in the prescription of a lifesaving medication. Of course, then they would have to practice like real physicians, like neurologists, for example!

A close parallel is in the cardiology with the drug Digitalis, which improves heart failure. Imagine that only 7.5 percent of cardiologists dared to prescribe it out of fear of side effects to their heart failure patients, letting them perish instead, because it too, like lithium, can have toxic effects if not prescribed with expertise!

Only 7 percent of psychiatrists in this country will prescribe lithium. That is not just ineptness—it is criminal!

GLOSSARY

ADLs. Routine activities performed on a daily basis, such as eating, bathing, dressing, toileting, walking, and continence.

adrenaline. Hormone secreted by adrenal gland in response to stress or anger.

aldosterone. A steroid hormone secreted by the adrenal gland that maintains salt and water balance.

allele. One of a number of alternative forms of a particular gene.

anterior temporal cortex. Part of cerebral cortex active in maintaining memory of objects, people, words, and facts.

apolipoprotein E (epsilon 4 allele, tau protein H1H1). A major cholesterol carrier supporting lipid transport.

basal ganglia. A group of subcortical nuclei responsible primarily for motor control, among other roles.

block reuptake of norepinephrine. A presynaptic neuron-making norepinephrine wants to pump it back into itself, but another molecule blocks the pump.

bradykinesia. Involuntary slowing down of movement, which usually is due to Parkinson's disease.

catechol-o-methyl transferase. An enzyme. Forms of this are used in the treatment of Parkinson's disease. Has beneficial effect on dopamine metabolism.

caudate. Also called striatum. A paired subcortical structure associated with basal ganglia and involved in memory and learning.

cholinesterase inhibitor. Chemicals that block the normal breakdown of the neurotransmitter, acetylcholine.

clozapine. A potent second-generation antipsychotic used to treat schizophrenia.

cortisol. An adrenal hormone that modulates stress responses.

default mode network (DMN). Refers to brain networks of interacting brain regions that are distinct from other brain networks.

demyelination. When the myelin sheath surrounding axons are damaged due to disease or trauma, which impairs conduction of the neuron's signal.

dopaminergic medications. They either facilitate the expression of dopamine or inhibit it. For example, some increase dopamine to treat Parkinson's disease; some decrease it to treat psychotic illnesses.

dopamine D4 receptor. A cousin to the DO receptor, relevant to the disease process of schizophrenia and Parkinson's disease.

dorsal anterior cingulate. Plays a role in reward-based decision-making, subserving cognition, and motor control.

dorsolateral prefrontal cortex. An area in the prefrontal cortex that plays a role in working memory.

dystonia. A neurological disorder in which muscle contractions are too sustained, resulting in abnormal fixed postures.

executive functions. A set of higher cognitive processes including attentional control, inhibitory control, working memory, reasoning, problem-solving, and planning.

GABA neurons. They produce gamma-amino-butyric acid, an inhibitory neurotransmitter.

glutamate neurons. They produce the excitatory neurotransmitter, glutamate.

glial cells. They closely accompany neurons providing for their optimal functioning.

inferior frontal cortex. Lateral surface of left cerebral hemisphere. Part of frontal lobe.

inflammatory cytokines. Molecules that are produced by activated macrophages, which increase neuro-inflammation.

intracellular signaling cascades. Signal relay pathways between neurons that ultimately influence gene expression.

Lewy bodies. Abnormal aggregates of protein that develop in nerve cells in Parkinson's disease and can cause dementia.

locus coeruleus. A grouping of neurons (nucleus) in the pons, part of the brain stem that produces noradrenaline.

monoamines. Another name for the main neurotransmitters, serotonin, dopamine, norepinephrine, and adrenaline.

movement disorder. Abnormal, involuntary bodily movements symptomatic of many neurological disorders.

negative neuroplastic changes. When due to trauma or neurological disease, the brain suffers reduction in reserve capacity and neurodegeneration.

neuroendocrine function. The mechanism by which the hypothalamus maintains normal regulation, in conjunction with the pituitary gland, of important bodily systems by releasing hormones into the blood.

neurotrophic signaling. A family of closely related proteins that control many aspects of development, survival, and functions of neurons.

nigrostriatal system. Modulates the extrapyramidal motor system. A dopaminergic pathway in the dorsal striatum.

noradrenergic neurons. Regulate the synthesis and release of noradrenaline.

Parkinson's disease. A disease of the nervous system marked by increasing tremor, muscular rigidity, and a slowing of movement associated with degeneration of the basal ganglia and dopamine deficiency.

parietal lobe. One of the four major lobes of the cerebral cortex.

posterior cingulate cortex. The posterior part of the cingulate cortex has an important role in cognition, but its specific nature is unclear.

pro-inflammatory cytokines. Examples are interleukin and tumor necrosis factor. When administered to humans, they produce fever, inflammation, tissue destruction, and in some cases shock and death.

psychosis. A severe mental disorder in which thought and emotions are so impaired that contact is lost with reality.

quetiapine. An atypical antipsychotic approved for the treatment of schizophrenia and bipolar disorder.

rigidity of muscles. In which they cannot normally relax. It can be associated with a number of disease states.

serotonin 5-HT2A receptor. An important serotonin receptor playing a role in MDD and suicidality.

serotonin transporter (reuptake pump). A membrane protein of the presynaptic neuron that pumps what would be wasted serotonin back into the neuron for subsequent use.

steroid. An organic compound utilized in the body for normal metabolic functions; it is subject to abuse if inappropriately ingested.

sympathetic nervous system. One of two main divisions of the autonomic nervous system; the other is the parasympathetic.

sympathetic activation. Can be overreactive, often associated with anxiety symptoms, cardiac symptoms, and hypertension.

visual hallucination. Visual phenomenon preoccupying the mind but not present in the external environment. There can be many causes.

visual processing deficits. A complex issue with eight types that often afflict people with schizophrenia and dyslexia.

white matter tracts. Bundles of axons that connect with different parts of the brain and transmit neuronal signals.

CHAPTER 21

Comorbidity

Comorbidity refers to medical conditions that are present simultaneously in a given patient—for example, diabetes and rheumatoid arthritis. Since therapy psychiatry treats only mental health problems, it's obvious those ethereal, psychological conditions cannot be subject to having comorbidities with real physical illnesses.

In the minds of therapy psychiatrists, they are responsible for treating the symptoms of mental problems, which requires specialized psychoanalytic approaches, particularly brilliant, incisive interpretations to attack the deep psychological conflicts buried in the id and superego. That is their area of expertise. They are not merely physicians; they are extremely sensitive, intuitive therapists who are concerned with the elevated problems of the psyche as compared to the more grubby preoccupations of physicians who treat mere physical disorders and problems.

Are therapy psychiatrists delusional? Are the human body and brain neatly sliced up into a mental part and a physical part? The therapy psychiatrists have a deep need to continue believing so. Otherwise they have to face the fact that they would have to begin making the effort to learn about the brain—not the id or the superego but the actual physical brain with its huge variety of neurotransmitters, receptors, messenger molecules, transcription factors, and genes. They can't even begin to contemplate that because it would commit them to becoming real physicians, like neurologists! (And that takes a lot of study and a lot of ongoing effort.)

In truth, there is no dividing line between mental and physical illnesses. There is actually no such thing as a mental illness except in the minds of therapy psychiatrists and the public they have influenced for a century! There are symptoms that are termed mental, but they do not come forth from the id and the superego. They come from the brain and other organs.

Many organs can generate mental symptoms—the thyroid gland, the adrenal gland, the parathyroid gland, the liver, the kidney, the bone marrow—and so can systemic illnesses like diabetes, fevers, dehydration, and electrolyte imbalance. Neurological diseases of the brain—stroke, myasthenia gravis, multiple sclerosis, and others—can also generate mental symptoms.)

The ABCs of Comorbidities

What does the adrenal gland have to do with attention deficit disorder? The adrenal glands are little mounds of physical tissue each kidney. Just looking at them, you know they are physical. They produce adrenaline, steroids, aldosterone, and cortisol. They don't look like they're mental. How could they have anything to do with attention deficit disorder, an obvious mental health problem? The association between them has therapy psychiatrists in a tizzy, setting off frenzied research to find a doppelganger of the adrenal gland in the id or the superego.

Children with tumors of the adrenal gland are three times more likely to also have a diagnosis of ADHD, a rate of 21 percent compared to 7 percent in children without adrenal tumors. Even though adrenal tumors are uncommon, the issue becomes important if the pediatrician is unaware of the association.

The prescription of stimulant medication for ADHD can put the nervous system into overdrive, resulting in a hypertensive crisis with possible stroke or the appearance of a large abdominal mass as the tumor grows and spreads. Following surgical removal of the tumor, the ADHD often will resolve. This is why a pediatrician can benefit from consulting with a brain psychiatrist who should be familiar with the important though rare association between adrenal tumors and ADHD. On the other hand, excessive caution in prescribing stimulant medications in those with severe ADHD can result in very impaired academic and social functioning, resulting ultimately in a legacy of failure and impoverishment in adulthood.[74]

What does the density of bones in children and adolescents have to with ADHD? Well, there is an association between reduced bone density and ADHD. Bones are obviously physical. Dogs bury them, and a club made of a long bone can knock you out. In this case, the factor to blame may be the medications prescribed for ADHD: stimulants.

Researchers evaluated 5,315 children and adolescents from 2005–2010. Their bone mineral density (BMD) was measured employing dual-energy x-ray absorptiometry.

Unfortunately, the study did not factor in medication dose, duration of use, or changes in therapy. Did the nonmedicated participants have a similar severity of ADHD compared to those on the stimulants? This is unclear. The authors advise, however, that clinicians should keep the issue of decreased BMD in mind and recommend nutritional counseling and other preventive measures. They recommend additional prospective studies. Again, provider expertise is essential.[75]

What possible connection could there be between cancer and depression? In cancer, of course, there is physical tissue, sometimes ounces or pounds of it, that has gone berserk. Maybe that's the

---

[74] "Adrenal gland tumors linked to ADHD diagnosis." Jessica Craig, *Clinical Psychiatry New Digital Network*, May 19, 2016.

[75] Howard J. T., Walick, K. S., Rivera, J. C. "Preliminary evidence of an association between ADHD medications and diminished bone health in children and adolescents," *J. Pediatr. Orthop.* 2015.

connection because people with mental health problems as a rule are berserk. Maybe that's the link!

Depression has been proposed as a predisposing factor for cancer. According to W. J. Brenda et al., writing in the ***Journal of the National Cancer Institute***, results of prior studies had been somewhat inconclusive because they measured depression at only a single time interval. Instead, in a large study investigating the relationship, they took a much more sophisticated approach. They enrolled 4,825 persons seventy-one years or older for their study, and they did periodic evaluations for depression starting at baseline (1988) and then at regular intervals over a six-year period.

They found that patients who had depressed moods over this six-year period had almost double the rate of cancers develop (HR 1.88) compared to those without depression. They speculated on possible explanations. A major one was that depressed patients have suppressed immune symptoms, deficiencies in cancer-fighting lymphocytes, and natural killer cell activity, probably related to a hypersensitive HPA axis and hypersecretion of cortisol.[76]

Two studies were conducted at Johns Hopkins Medical School, and the results were released on July 18, 2012. Individuals with serious mental illness were found to be 2.6 times more likely to develop cancer than the general population. They were two to three times more likely to die prematurely, 4.5 times more likely to develop lung cancer, 3.5 times more like to develop colorectal cancer, and three times more likely to develop breast cancer, and these cancers developed at an average younger age of forty-two to forty-three years.

The researchers questioned whether the patients received appropriate screening for cancer, and it was recommended that mental health providers and primary care physicians must work together to promote screening.[77]

---

[76] "Chronically Depressed Mood and Cancer Risk in Older Persons." Prenda W. J. et al. *Journal of the National Cancer Institute* (1998) 90 (24): 1888–1893).

[77] "Cancer and Injuries More Likely in People with Serious Mental Illness," Gail L. Daumit, MD, MHS, *Psychiatric Services Study*, July 18, 2012.)

This author has to guffaw—tragically—that therapy psychiatrists pay any attention to issues of screening for grubby physical illnesses like cancer. What's important is imparting to the possibly cancer-ridden patient a brilliant, incisive interpretation to dissolve a ferocious deep conflict in the Id or Superego.

In general, although cancer care today provides state-of-the-art biomedical treatment, it fails to address the psychological and psychosocial problems associated with the illness. This failure can compromise the effectiveness of health care and adversely affect the health of cancer patients by causing additional suffering and weakening adherence to prescribed treatments.

Although the majority of cancer patients have normal psychological functioning, approximately 29–43 percent have an overlay of significant psychological distress in addition to the direct suffering caused by the cancer.

Data from the President's Cancer Panel in 2003 and 2004 disclosed cancer survivors of all ages reported many health providers treating cancer still do not consider psychosocial support an integral component of quality cancer care and may fail to recognize, adequately treat, or refer for depression, anger, and stress in cancer survivors.[78] These providers may be humanoids, believing human beings are actually robots who do not experience emotions!

A number of studies have shown some oncology providers are inattentive to psychosocial problems, and they don't think of referring their patients and wouldn't know who to refer to anyway. Fat chance they'd ever diagnose major depression! (What the hell? You have cancer. You might as well feel hopeless or even suicidal. What's the difference?)

---

[78] *Cancer Care for the Whole Patient.* Editors Nancy E. Adler, et al. Institute of Medicine, Washington, D.C.: National Academies Press (US), 2008.

Diabetes

A large scientific study was completed in Germany in 2014 to determine if there is an association between depression and metabolic outcome. They studied poor control of blood sugar levels and the measurement (HbA1c) in younger people, ages eighteen to twenty-one, with type 1 diabetes. They found 43 percent of the male diabetics and 33 percent of the females demonstrated at least one symptom of depression. About 5 percent had a full syndrome of major depression. HbA1c levels were elevated (indicating poorer response to diabetes treatment if the following symptoms of depression were present: psycho-motor agitation or retardation, poor appetite or overeating, insomnia, and lethargy.[79]

Dementia

There have been two well-designed scientific studies evaluating the association of depression and dementia, chiefly Alzheimer's disease. The first followed 2,488 individuals who had repeated assessment for symptoms of depression from the start of the study to year five. All of them were free of dementia over that period. The individuals with severe depression who did not improve were twice as likely to go on to develop dementia than those with milder depression.

The great majority of patients were not receiving antidepressant medication. The researchers recommended depressed elderly people be monitored over a long-time span. (Fat chance. There are practically no psychiatrists who like to treat elderly patients. Their ids and superegos are spent entities with nary a deeply buried unconscious conflict worth bothering with.)

If one is or has an elderly relative who is depressed (and the family might have to make the diagnosis since the family doctor probably

---

[79] "Association between HbA1c and depressive symptoms in young adults with early-onset type 1 diabetes." B. Christina et al. *Science Direct*, January 30, 2015. German Center for Diabetes Research.

won't), it may be best to seek a consultation at a high-quality medical school hospital. Usually each state has at least one.[80]

The second study followed 3,325 individuals, ages seventy-four to eighty-eight years, for ten years, periodically evaluating for symptoms of both dementia and depression. Of them, 434 individuals went on to develop dementia. The risk was 50 percent greater for depressed in comparison to nondepressed individuals.[81]

Depression, Diabetes, and Dementia

A very large study involving a total of 2,454,532 adults including 477,133 (19.4 percent) with depression and 223,174 (9.1 percent) with diabetes and 95,691 (3.9 percent) with both, was run in Denmark from January 1, 2007, through December 31, 2013.

At the start of the study, all subjects were free of dementia. Over the course of the study, 59,663 participants developed dementia (2.4 percent). Of those, 6,466 (10.8 percent) had diabetes, 15,729 (26.4 percent) had depression, and 4,022 (6.7 percent) had both.

The hazard ratio (the chance of developing dementia) was 1.83 for depression (nearly double the rate of those without depression, and 1.20 higher than those with diabetes. In other words, each disorder is an independent risk factor for dementia, though depression (a mere mental health problem) results in more risk than diabetes (a real physical disease).

How could that be so? What do those deeply buried conflicts in the id have to do with a physical substance like glucose? (Therapy psychiatrists have repudiated the findings of this study!)

A central finding of this huge study is that those with depression and diabetes develop dementia at a rate greater than the sum of each disease separately. In addition, individuals with depression develop

---

[80] "Trajectories of Depressive Symptoms in Older Adults and Risk of Dementia." Kaup, Allison R., et al, *JAMA Psychiatry*, 2016: 73(5), 525–531.

[81] Mirza, S.S. et al. "Ten-year trajectories of depressive symptoms and risk of dementia, a population-based study." *The Lancet Psychiatry*. Published Online, April 29, 2016.)

diabetes five years earlier than those without depression. Dually affected individuals have a 5 percent chance of developing dementia before the age of sixty-five—far earlier than the typical age of onset.

The researchers considered the above situation from a public health perspective. The expense of chronic disease at younger ages is what they term *the disease burden*. As good citizens and well-intentioned researchers, they recommended developing screening and interventions to improve the quality of treatment of depression and diabetes in the riskiest subgroup of patients by integrating medical and psychiatric care. That's a laugh—a tragic laugh.

The therapy psychiatrists are off in their own mental health care system, and they can't be bothered by a physical issue like diabetes. It has nothing to do with what's important from their vantage point. At any rate, a brilliant psychological interpretation is attacking a deep conflict in the id might cure the diabetes.

Cardiovascular Disease

According to therapy psychiatry, depression is a mere mental health problem. Most depressed people could just snap themselves out of it if they had any backbone at all. If, due to some deficiency in their characters, they don't have the capacity to do that, they should consult with therapy psychiatrists who will snap them out of it by issuing brilliant psychological interpretations that will dissolve deep unconscious conflicts in the id and superego in identical fashion for cardiovascular disease as for diabetes. (It may take two or more years.)

Few depressed older adults receive effective treatment in the primary care setting.[82] Primary care physicians are extraordinarily busy, so they must prioritize their time. Since therapy-psychiatry affirms depression is a mere mental health problem, their precious time must be spent diagnosing and treating physical illnesses. There

---

[82] Unuzer, J., et all, "Collaborative-care management of late-life depression in the primary care setting." *JAMA*, 2002; 288 (22): 2836-45.

is no time to inquire about the symptoms of depression, particularly since the diagnosis can't be confirmed by specific laboratory testing.

Therefore, unless a patient is so extremely depressed they can barely move or speak (psycho-motor retardation), the diagnosis of depression is never made. And for the rare conscientious primary care physician who actually asks about the symptoms of depression, they probably have the illness themselves (albeit treated). And even if they may refer to their favorite mental health professional, or if it should be a psychiatrist, the odds are 70–80 percent it will be a therapy psychiatrist.

What if depression isn't diagnosed or treated competently? In findings from the impact study of Dr. Quyyumi, a researcher, it was pointed out that depression may have more significance than previously known for increasing the risk of heart attack and stroke.[83] The Impact Intervention Trial found when depression was diagnosed and treated competently, either with an antidepressant medication and/or psychotherapy, the risk of heart attack decreased by 48 percent (nearly a 50 percent reduction in the occurrence of heart attacks—and a similar reduction in strokes).

In comparison to matched patients who received no treatment for depression, Dr. Quyyumi emphasized, "We need to recognize that the incidence of depression is high in this population, and if depression is present, the outcome is a lot worse."

An examination for depression need only take a few minutes, for example, by having patients fill out the one-page BDI-II.

If the depression was not diagnosed early and on a timely basis, it was too late to prevent the cardiovascular disease that followed soon after the onset of depression. This is one reason the so-called mental health care system is so pathetic. It fails to diagnose and treat depression competently, setting up tens of thousands of people for

---

[83] Summarized by Tori Rodriguez, MA, LPC, summarized in *Psychiatry Advisor*, February 1, 2016, "The Link Between Depression and Cardiovascular Disease: The Findings of the Impact Study in a 2014 Issue of the *Journal of Behavioral Medicine*."

a significantly greater risk of both heart attacks and strokes. This is really malpractice writ large!

Another study reviewed the relationship between depression and cardiovascular disease (CVD).[84] Patients with CVD have three times the risk of developing depression symptoms, which significantly worsen the prognosis for both cardiovascular and noncardiovascular outcomes.

Results showed a direct correlation between elevated BDI scores (measuring clinical depressive symptoms) and elevation of multiple biological markers for CVD. How can depression, a mental health problem, affect biological markers for heart disease? (Therapy psychiatry researchers have temporarily been thrown into a tizzy, insisting that depression, a direct result of deep psychological conflict in the id and superego, must have a nonphysical mechanisms for elevating the biological markers. They are contemplating numerous possible psychoanalytic explanations.)

Although there is more research needed, there is evidence that depression mediates CVD through several physical mechanisms: activation of the hypothalamic pituitary axis, an imbalance between the sympathetic and parasympathetic branches of the autonomic nervous system, stimulation of oxidative stress and inflammatory signaling, and acceleration of metabolic processes promoting vascular dysfunction and arteriosclerosis.

Researchers carefully investigated the relationship between depressive symptoms in 965 individuals who had not yet been diagnosed with CVD. Symptoms of depression were assessed using the Beck Depression Inventory II (BDI-II).

Results showed the higher the BDI scores, the higher the biological markers for CVD, higher AIX, C-reactive protein (CRP), as well as lower SEVR and glutathione levels. The more severe the depressive symptoms, the worse the vascular stiffening and inflammation.

Arshed A. Quyyumi, MD, professor of medicine at Emory

---

[84] Tori Rodriguez, MA, LPC, Psychiatry Advisor, Feb. 01, 2016. Study appearing in The Journal of the American College of Cardiology.

University School of Medicine, pointed out none of the subjects in the study had CVD at the start. He stated, "We were basically looking at this well before the symptoms of CVD—whether early symptoms of depression were associated with early changes associated with heart disease."

He added, "The participants had no recognition that they were depressed, and even at this very early stage, all these arterial abnormalities were present."

(Dr. Quyyumi is an internist, not a psychiatrist. While he and many like him are doing serious research on the symptoms and disabilities wrought by clinical depression, therapy psychiatrists remain preoccupied with issues focused on the id and superego.)

A third study was summarized by Laura Stiles, assistant editor of ***Psychiatry Advisor.***[85] The results of the original study were presented at the 2016 American College of Cardiology's Annual Scientific Session and Expo in Chicago. This study drew the conclusion that prompt, effective treatment of depression appears to improve the risk of poor heart health, according to Heidi May, PhD—a cardiovascular epidemiologist with the Intermountain Medical Center Heart Institute. The researchers there examined 7,550 patients over a course of two years. The patients were forty-five to sixty-nine years old, and 70 percent were women.

The frequency of serious cardiovascular events was approximately 50 percent higher for those who were depressed or became depressed than for those who had no depression, or whose depression went into remission. The authors also concluded that changes in depression symptoms may cause immediate physiological changes in the body that can cause major cardiac events in the short term.[86]

---

[85] April 5, 2016, "Can Effectively Treating Depression Reduce Cardiovascular or Risk?"

[86] May HT, Brunisholz K, Horne B, et al. Can Effective Treatment of Depression Reduce Future Cardiovascular Risk? Presented at 2016 American College of Cardiology (ACC) 65th Annual Scientific Session and Expo, April 2–4, 2016; Chicago, Illinois.

Immunity

Clinical Depression is generally precipitated by significant stressors, and once a full-blown episode has occurred, it is one of the most stress-inducing illnesses known.[87] This study was published in the ***Journal of Neuroscience***. Research in mice was meant to simulate the effects of severe stress in humans. It was the first study to establish a relationship between lasting stress and disruption of short-term memory. The mice were taught to recall the location of an escape hole in a maze they had repeatedly mastered. They were then exposed to an aggressive intruder mouse. The dominance by an alpha mouse was meant to mimic chronic psychosocial stress in humans. The experimental mice who were exposed to the intruder had a difficult time remembering the location of the escape hole. They didn't recall it in contrast to the unstressed mice who readily remembered it.

Neural progenitor cells that proliferated in the stressed mice remained abnormal for up to a month after the stressor occurred. The researchers concluded that the memory problems appearing after the stress were directly linked to inflammation and impairments in the immune system.

According to John Sheridan, PhD, associate director of Ohio State's Institute for Behavioral Medicine Research, stress releases immune cells from the bone marrow, and those cells can traffic to the brain areas associated with neuronal activation in response to stress. He said, "They're being called to the brain, to the center of memory."[88]

Another report, "Psychological Success and the Human Immune System: A Meta-Analytic Study of 30 Years of Inquiry,[89] reviewed three hundred empirical articles describing a relationship

---

[87] "Chronic Stress Impacts Immune system, Inhibits Memory." Laura Stiles, assistant editor, *Psychiatric Advisor*, March 2, 2016.

[88] McKim DB, Niraula A., Tarr AJ, Wohleb ES, Sheridan JF, Godbout JP. Neuroinflammatory Dynamics Underlie Memory Impairment after Repeated Social Defeat. *J. Neurosci.* 2016; doi: 10.1523/jneurosci. 2394-15.2016.

[89] Psychological Stress and the Human Immune System: A Meta-Analytic Study of 30 Years of Inquiry, Suzanne C. Cederstrom and Gregory E. Miller.

between psychological stress and parameters of the immune system in human participants. This particular focus of interest is termed *psychoneuroimmunology.* The researchers stated these multiple studies have convincingly established stressful experiences confer vulnerability for the onset of diseases and more adverse outcomes by how they impact the immune system.

Neuroscience is working out the rather complex mechanisms by which stress, especially chronic stress does this. A principle mechanism operates via excessive expression of inflammatory molecules, particularly cytokines. Chronic stress elicits the prolonged secretion of cortisol which causes white blood cells to mount a counter-regulatory response[90] by downregulating their cortisol receptors. This, in turn, reduces the cells' capacity to respond to anti-inflammatory signals, allowing excessive levels of cytokine-mediated inflammatory responses. Such excessive inflammatory processes in turn predispose people to the outbreak of diseases and contribute to more adverse outcomes of them, which in turn elevates morbidity and mortality. A wide variety of disease states are influenced by this process: multiple sclerosis, rheumatoid arthritis, coronary artery disease, asthma, allergy, etc. But guess what? The so-called mental health problems, so coined by therapy-psychiatry, operates in terms of stress dynamics in identical fashion to the real physical diseases!

A list of potential stressors (not all inclusive): any serious disease, surgical procedures, inappropriate or incomplete treatment for disease, smoking, not following or refusing appropriate treatment, poverty, illiteracy, academic failure, underachievement at school, educational maladjustment with discord with teachers, unemployment, threat of job loss, change of job, stressful work schedule, discord with boss or workmates, difficult conditions at work, homelessness, inadequate housing, discord with neighbors, lodgers, and landlords, low income, insufficient social insurance and welfare support, foreclosures, problems with creditors, empty nest syndrome, problem with adjustment to retirement, problems with living alone, exclusion

---

[90] Ibid.

or rejection on basis of personal characteristics such as unusual physical appearance, illness, or behavior, target of discrimination, disappearance or death of family members, disruption of family by separation and divorce, other stressful life events affecting the family or household, illness, martial estrangement, dependent relative, high expressed emotional level in family, inadequate financial support, inadequate or distorted family communication, unwanted pregnancy.

Other Medical and Metabolic Disorders

A very comprehensive study of the relationship of mental illness to the onset of physical illnesses was conducted over a ten-year period[91] (January 1, 2001–December 31, 2011). The researchers' objective was to investigate associations of sixteen temporally identified mental disorders with the subsequent onset of ten chronic physical conditions. They conducted eighteen face-to-face interviews with each of 47,609 individuals in seventeen countries. They assessed for the lifetime prevalence of both mental and physical illness.

Most associations between the mental disorders and the subsequent diagnosis of physical disorders were statistically significant. For example, the presence of mood (unipolar or bipolar) disorders, anxiety disorders, and substance abuse disorders along with the increasing severity of their symptoms was proportional to the frequency of onset and associated worsening of the physical illnesses. The range of increases in physical illness was 1.4 to 6.5 times greater than in individuals not having mental disorders.

They summarized, the greater the amount and frequency of the symptoms of mental illness, the greater the odds of developing severe physical illnesses. They point out how the deleterious effects of mental disorders on physical health start early in the course of mental illnesses, which usually have an earlier onset than physical

---

[91] "Association of Mental Disorders with Subsequent Chronic Physical Conditions," Scott, Karen, M, PhD et al. *JAMA Psychiatry*, Published online December 23, 2015.

disorders in general. They urge treatment of all mental disorders should optimally incorporate attention to physical health and health behaviors with this parallel focus on physical health commencing at the initiation of mental health care treatment, which does not occur currently.

They also recommend that primary care physicians be more proactive in diagnosing and treating their mental health patients. (Welcome, again to the treacherous dichotomy, in which mental illness receives mental treatment in the mental health care system with little or no attention to matters of physical health. In the physical health care system, primary physicians either ignore their patients' mental health symptoms or—under the influence of therapy psychiatry—refer them to a wide range of mental health resources.

The mentally ill are living ten to twenty-five years less. Year after year, these stunning incongruities continue. This is a manifestation of society's dysfunction and anosognosia.

This author does not disagree with Dr. Nasrallah's assessment and must point out the fault is not largely with society, but with psychiatry. As long as psychiatry identifies the illnesses they are responsible for as mental illnesses, they will always be thought of as second-class mental health problems. There must come forth from some authoritative source that what are identified as mental health problems should no longer be framed in that degrading matter. Instead, they are physical brain diseases like Parkinson's disease and multiple sclerosis. When they are seen in exactly the same physical category—only then will the discrimination stop!

HPV (Human Papilloma Virus)

You feel a little depressed? So what? It's just an emotion and can't harm you! However, it does apparently invigorate viruses! The presence of depression and its attendant stress may play a role in whether an infected woman can get rid of her infection or not.[92] Lead investigator Anna-Barbara Moscicki, MD, FAAP, chief of the Division of Adolescent and Young Adult Medicine and Professor of Pediatrics at the University of California, Los Angeles School of Medicine reviewed data on a group of 333 women researchers had been studying for their research since 2000. They had been an average age of nineteen when they were enrolled in the study.

Throughout the study period, every six months, the level of the HPV was measured in laboratory. At the age of twenty-eight, they filled out extensive questionnaires assessing degrees of depression and stress. The end point of the study was whether the women had persistence of the virus in their bodies or had become free of infection. The women who were depressed or perceived themselves as having a lot of stress were more likely to remain infected. Dr. Moscicki said the study suggests that reduction of stress (and depression is triggered by stress and greatly augments it) may help them clear their infections.

Neurological Disorders

Neurological illnesses are the other main grouping of diseases that affect the brain. They are categorized as real physical illnesses treated by real physicians (neurologists). There is no such thing as a therapy neurologist. The actual brain is the organ they concentrate on—both to understand its physical dysfunctions and the medical treatments, which include a wide variety of pharmacological agents.

There is almost certainly not a living neurologist who has been able to locate the id and superego in the brain, and this is not just because they would have absolutely no interest in looking for them. By definition, all neurologists are brain neurologists. They are the first providers to evaluate patients for neurological symptoms, although many referrals come from internists and family physicians. Patients are evaluated by the neurologists first, and then possibly referred to

---

[92] *Psychiatry Advisor*, May 5, 2016. A summary of a presentation at the Pediatric Academic Society's 2016 Meeting in Baltimore, Maryland, May 2016.

associated nonmedical therapist (physical therapists, occupational therapists, physical medicine, rehabilitation specialists, etc.). This is the exact opposite of what occurs in the mental health care system—in which the brain psychiatrist is often last in the link of providers, if ever seen in consultation at all!

Migraine

Anyone who has experienced a severe migraine has been initiated into the particular type of suffering it can cause. Overwhelming nausea, a hammering, throbbing head, a need to get to a quiet, dark place. Of course, the more severe cases can be highly recurrent. Thank heavens, there are treatments, but they only work well in about 50 percent of patients, leading to significant pain reduction for at least two hours.

Richard B. Lipton, MD, of the Albert Einstein College of Medicine in New York City, analyzed the results from the American Migraine Prevalence and Prevention study survey database. Of the 8,333 patients, 4,666 (56 percent) had an inadequate response. The three major causes for this were a condition called allodynia (in which neurons are hypersensitive to minor pain stimuli, i.e., even touching the skin results in pain), failure to take anti-migraine medications as prescribed, and depression. The recommendation is physicians should assess patients for factors that may predict inadequate response in order to improve the likelihood of rapid and consistent migraine relief. (Want to make a bet? Probably migraine patients are never checked for clinical depression!)

Epilepsy

An epileptic seizure is the result of a temporary physiologic dysfunction of the brain caused by an abnormal, self-limited, and hypersynchronous electrical discharge of cortical neurons.[93] Epilepsy generally is a chronic group of disorders that are typically

[93] *Merritt's Neurology*, thirteenth edition, 468.

unpredictable and unprovoked. Except for one type of epilepsy, simple partial seizures, consciousness is always impaired.

The physician specialist most knowledgeable about the various types of epilepsy and the broad spectrum of appropriate treatments is the board-certified neurologist. Interestingly, even though both neurology and psychiatry receive certification by a common organization, the American Board of Psychiatry and Neurology, there is little overlap in their fields of study. This diminishes with time since the bulk of psychiatrists begin building therapy-psychiatry practices in which issues of brain structures, mechanisms, and functions are of little interest to them. Brain psychiatrists are much more likely to display an interest in neurological disorders and treatments and maintain some degree of communications with their neurological colleagues.

A few enlightened neurologists (there aren't many) are aware of the psychiatric comorbidities accompanying seizure disorders. On the whole, neurological practice emphasizing working up and treating the seizure disorders does not even assess for possible comorbid psychiatric illnesses, which are grossly underdiagnosed and dramatically undertreated! And yet epileptic patients have significantly greater symptomatic burden than people without epilepsy: 17.4 percent MDD, 22.8 percent anxiety disorders, 34 percent combined mood and anxiety symptoms, and 25 percent suicidal ideation.[94] (Five percent of epileptic patients eventually commit suicide, a level equal to psychiatric disorders). The professors strongly assert that comprehensive care of the epileptic patient requires attention to the psychological and social consequences of epilepsy and control of seizures.

The neurologist, by neglecting to display any interest in comorbid psychiatric disorders in epilepsy patients, is almost certainly worsening the prognosis for successful treatment of the seizure disorder. The two

---

[94] "Psychiatric Disorders Associated with Epilepsy." Fahad Salih Algreeshah, MD (Head of Neurology, King Saud Medical Center and Selim RLS Benbadis, MD, Professor, Dept. of Neurological, University of South Florida College of Medicine.

categories of disorders tend to feed off each other, one exacerbating the other and vice versa.

Untreated psychiatric illnesses result in more frequent hospitalizations, higher treatment costs, and a greater percentage of drug-resistant seizures and reductions in seizure remission rates. The most common psychiatric disorder in epileptic patients is MDD, but a whole spectrum can occur: bipolar disorder, panic disorder, other anxiety disorders, obsessive-compulsive disorder, and substance abuse disorders.

It is a shame, but therapy psychiatry, by maintaining its preoccupation with so-called psychological structures like the id and the superego, and being largely and totally ignorant of the biologically based multiple physical brain abnormalities that cause the major psychiatric illnesses, are unable to communicate with neurologists. If they were conversant with the actual physical (real) brain, there would be a common language between them and profitable discussion that the two categories of illness actually share many related brain pathologies:[95] decreased levels of serotonin and norepinephrine, abnormalities of their transport or postsynaptic binding, abnormal activity of GABA and dopamine, aberrant nerve regeneration and glial proliferation, and structural abnormalities in the limbic system, especially the hippocampus. Six MRI studies have documented that patients with MDD have excessive loss of gray matter.

In other words, neurological disorders and the major psychiatric disorders are locked together in a single unified brain. The two should not be separated; they exist conjointly and interactively. It is therapy psychiatry that perpetuates the separation into the so-called mental health care system and the general medical (physical illness) system. The unnecessary magnification of illness, suffering, and disabilities on the backs of millions of patients is intolerable. It must end. The gripping fingers of therapy-psychiatry must be pulled off the necks of those they call mentally ill, so these unfortunate individuals will know

---

95 "Managing Psychiatric Illness in Patients with Epilepsy." Sowmya C. Puvvada, MD, et al. *Current Psychiatry,* May 13, 2014, (5): 30–38.

they are not mentally ill and can be included in the general physical health care system.

Once there are sufficient brain psychiatrists who can collaborate with neurologists, neurologists can be taught to recognize psychiatric illness and make appropriate referral to a brain psychiatrist. The brain psychiatrist, like the neurologist, will use sophisticated pharmacology, will understand potential drug interactions between medications for neurological disorders and psychiatric disorders, and like the neurologist, will be expert in utilizing physical treatments such as vagus nerve stimulation, transcranial magnetic stimulation, deep-brain stimulation, and in the most dire cases of mood disorders, competently administered electroconvulsive therapy.

The key will be collaboration between the neurologist and the brain psychiatrist since they both are expert in the one brain. That brain must be treated in the same medical system!

Some enlightened physicians actually simulated such a system, but in primary care[96] (which could serve as a model for the neurologist and brain psychiatrist collaboration in the treatment of neurological and psychiatric disorders.) The objective of their study was to compare the effectiveness of a multifaceted intervention in patients with depression in primary care with the usual care they would have received.

Over a twelve-month period, collaboration between the primary care physician and a consulting psychiatrist by scheduling appointments with both providers built in, so to speak, while the nonintervention patients continued usual care for depression with the primary care physician. Seventy-four percent of the intervention patients showed 50 percent or greater improvement on the Symptom Checklist-90 Depressive Symptom Scale compared to 43 percent for the usual treatment patients (a 32 percent difference). Those who had more severe depressions had the most relative improvement. This author is assuming the psychiatrists collaborating with the primary

[96] Katon W., et. al, "Collaborative management to achieve treatment guidelines. Impact on depression in primary care." *Abstract, JAMA*, April 5, 1995; 273 (13); 1026–31.

care physicians were more medically oriented, most likely brain psychiatrists.

Other neurological diseases which are very often intertwined with the mental health problems (so designated by therapy psychiatry) are stroke, Parkinson's disease, and multiple sclerosis. Maybe one day, therapy psychiatry—by some manipulation of their thinking—will explain how such real (physical) brain illnesses should have any relationship with the id and superego causing mental illness.

What can a simple mental health problem have anything to do with a stroke? Obviously an illness can physically damage (real) brain tissue. In the former, you can just snap out of, the latter quite obviously not!

Abhishek Srivastava, et al., of the Center for Physical Medicine and Rehabilitation at the Ambani Hospital in Bangalore, India,[97] conducted a study to evaluate the prevalence of operationally defined depressive disorder (ICD-10) in chronic stroke subjects to determine the relationship of poststroke depression (PSD) with disability. They identified stroke as a major public health problem that results in disabilities of 24–54 percent, according to several studies.

According to several studies, poststroke depression has a prevalence rate of 18–61 percent in stroke survivors. However, it remains largely undiagnosed and/or undertreated in spite of its association with more cognitive impairment, greater risk of falls, worse rehabilitation outcomes, and increased disability and mortality. The researchers admitted stroke patients to their facility after they had received treatment at peripheral hospitals—generally for at least three months. Their ages ranged from sixteen to sixty-five.

Out of a total of 167 patients, they selected fifty-one patients who were most suitable for the study, those who were poststroke an average of 467 days. Of the fifty-one patients ultimately included in the study, eighteen were diagnosed as depressed as per ICD-10 criteria. Surprisingly, none of these patients had received any specific

---

97 "Poststroke depression: Prevalence and relationship with disability in chronic stroke survivors," Ann Indian Acad. Neurol., April–June 2010; 13 (2): 123–127.

treatment for depression. (And this was after a year and a half after the initial stroke! This author is definitely not surprised. As long as psychiatry labels depression a mental versus a real physical illness, nonpsychiatric physicians just ignore it!)

The stroke patients with major depression were compared to the stroke patients who were not clinically depressed. Those with depression were worse off on every count: more impaired cognition, balance, walking ability, and ADLs. The researchers stated, "A major concern is that none of the depressed patients were on any antidepressant treatment. Patients not having depression had better odds of returning to work and a better functional recovery."

They pointed out the diagnosis of PSD was made by psychiatrists following operationally defined guidelines, demonstrating the need for multidisciplinary teams in rehabilitation. They discussed the advantages of collaboration as reducing suffering, promoting more effective treatment of stroke survivors, and reducing costs. (This author knows little about how psychiatry is practiced in India. Presumably, therapy psychiatrists are busily uncovering id and superego issues in the wealthiest neighborhoods in India. We know for sure that there is at least one brain psychiatrist in India—the one who worked collaboratively with the researchers who conducted this study).

Parkinson's Disease

Parkinson's disease (PD) is a neurodegenerative disorder caused by the loss of dopaminergic neurons in the midbrain, which results in dysfunction of the nigrostriatal system producing alterations in movement such as tremor, bradykinesia (slowed movement), rigidity, and postural abnormalities. PD is characterized as a movement disorder, but depression occurs frequently in this population with a prevalence of 30–40 percent.[98] With some minor editing, the following is taken verbatim from a Michael J. Fox Foundation research report:

> When facing a diagnosis of Parkinson's disease, it is understandable to feel anxious or depressed. But mood disorders such as anxiety and depression are real clinical symptoms of Parkinson's, just as rigidity and tremor.

How Can I Get Help for Depression or Anxiety?

MDD often accompanies Parkinson's disease. It could require its own individual treatment. Ask your neurologist or primary care physician about this. Also, you can google a self-administered rating scale for major depression.

Of course, the Fox report must emphasize that clinical depression is real and adds that it is important to remember that clinical depression and anxiety are underdiagnosed in people with Parkinson's and that they are symptoms of disease—not character flaws. Such a claim is very wounding to therapy psychiatrists who deeply believe there are such character flaws that require deep psychoanalytic psychotherapy through which their brilliant, concise interpretations attack the deeply buried conflicts causing such character flaws, which will thus be alleviated. The issue of therapy psychiatrists accepting patients with serious Parkinson's disease is somewhat moot because they are considered too grubbily physical and lacking the insight that would enable deep, incisive psychoanalytic interpretations to have any benefit at all.

A small study, "The Impact of Depression on Survival of

---

[98] "Depression in Parkinson's Disease: Health risks, etiology, and treatment options," Frisim G. Pasquale, et al, Neuropsychiatr. Dis. Treat. Feb 4, 2008 (1): 81–89.

Parkinson's Disease Patients: A Five-Year Study,"[99] was conducted in Brazil to evaluate the survival rate in a cohort of Parkinson's disease patients with and without depression. They entered, after appropriate screening, sixty-three Parkinson's disease patients and monitored them for five years (2003–2008). Of these, twenty-one were diagnosed with depression. The cumulative survival rate was 83 percent, with nine deaths: five in the depressed group and four in the nondepressed group. The depressed group showed a higher rate of mortality than the nondepressed group.

The hazard ratio (HR) for deaths of PD patients was 2.17 times higher in the depressed subgroup. In their discussion, the researchers note Parkinson's disease has a threefold increase in mortality compared with non-PD elderly populations. They also note another study that observed a chronically depressed population for six years and found a 41 percent increase in mortality compared to nondepressed subjects. The results of their eleven-year study were consistent with another study that also found the mortality for depressed PD patients was 2.66 higher than nondepressed PD patients. "These results are pointing in the same direction."

They also reviewed a more recent study in a large elderly population that presented convincing data with regards to the direct relationship between mortality and the severity of the depressive symptoms, which they term a dose-response relationship. They discuss mechanisms by which depression increases mortality. Depression complicates the course of neurological disorders. A series of pathophysiological cascades with cytokines (IL6, alpha TNF) and lower levels of protective factors (BDNF, IGF1) are triggered by clinical depression. Inflammatory states are a likely cause of higher mortality and neurodegeneration. They point out, "All these factors also are present in Parkinson's disease."

If there is such an overlapping of biological pathologies between Parkinson's and major depression, by what process of cognitive

---

[99] Silberman, Claudia D. et al. *Journal Braileiro de Psiquiatria*. vol. 62, no. 1 Rio de Janeiro, 2013.

pathology can therapy psychiatrists, who probably admit Parkinson's disease is physical, simultaneously proclaim MDD is mental? (Their bible is *The Diagnostic and Statistical Manual of Mental Disorders.*) Actually, there is an answer: Therapy psychiatrists suffer from having an archaic dogma in which they are beholden to near-delusional ideas that diseases that are proven by neuroscience to be biologically based. However, they are really not. Instead, they are conceptualized in terms of a more or less distorted set of psychoanalytic-religious beliefs, still held as in ancient times, before the advent of modern scientific research.

The final article, "Depression in Parkinson's Disease: Health risks, etiology, and treatment options,[100] stated right up front in the abstract that although 30–40 percent of PD patients suffer from depression, only a small percentage (about 20 percent) receive any treatment for it. As a result, many PD patients suffer with reduced health-related quality of life. Patients with Parkinson's disease often overlook symptoms of depression and focus instead on their motor deficit symptoms. (It's no surprise they overlook their depressive symptoms because everyone else does!) Besides, it is a difficult diagnosis to make, requiring a systematic approach. Therefore, the authors strongly urge physicians to screen for depression. (This is easy—just have them complete the BDI or similar scale). But doctors don't!

Depression adds an additional burden of symptoms to the motor symptoms: a more negative outlook, hopelessness, impaired motivation, and capacity to follow through on the treatment for PD, reduced energy, anhedonia, more stigma, impaired cognition, increased pain and bodily discomfort, and reduced social drive and social isolation.

Imaging studies have demonstrated differences between PD patients who have depression and those who don't. PET scans demonstrate metabolic abnormalities in both the caudate and inferior

---

[100] "Depression in Parkinson's Disease: Health risks etiology, and treatment options," Pasquale G. Frisina, et al, *Neuropsychiatr De Treat* Feb. 4, 2008, (1): 81–91.

frontal cortices as compared to nondepressed PD patients, as well as lower metabolic activity in the prefrontal cortex.[101]

Treatment requires a high level of pharmacological expertise. A class of antidepressant medications, tricyclic antidepressants like imipramine (150–250 mg/day) or others have a dual benefit, but also potential severe side effects if prescribed by an inexperienced practitioner. (Most therapy psychiatrists have virtually no expertise and never prescribe tricyclics. If one does, be sure to go to the website of a good medical school to read up on the drug).

Tricyclics alleviate the symptoms of clinical depression and can improve the motor symptoms of Parkinson's disease (What? How can a mental drug for a mental health problem also work for a real physical disease like Parkinson's disease?) The tricyclics block the reuptake of the neurotransmitter norepinephrine, which is linked to Parkinson's disease as well as depression. It leads to improved dopamine levels within the basal ganglia by boosting noradrenergic neurons in the locus coeruleus in PD patients.

Because therapy psychiatrists are generally so limited in pharmacological expertise, they will prescribe SSRIs (selective serotonin reuptake inhibitors) if they accept a patient with PD. This class of drugs, if prescribed carefully and at adequate dosage, can alleviate depression but not the motor symptoms of PD. In some cases, SSRIs may worsen the motor symptoms. Unfortunately, there are not enough brain psychiatrists to go around. Most patients with PD are left to wither and suffer much more than necessary. Neither they nor their families are aware of why the degree of suffering is occurring and have nowhere to turn for competent treatment.

A few competent brain psychiatrists, generally at the well-known medical schools, are capable of competently diagnosing PD and treating it. There is a wide therapeutic armamentarium. The tricyclic antidepressants, MAOI inhibitors, dopaminergic drugs, and even

---

[101] "Depression in Parkinson's Disease: Health risks, etiology, treatment options."

electroconvulsive therapy, which like tricyclic antidepressants, might have dual benefit.

The researchers plead that patients with PD receive timely treatment, requiring accurate diagnosis of depression and expert focused treatment (fat chance for the great majority of these patients!)

Another mental health problem that occurs in PD is Parkinson's disease psychosis.[102] The main symptom is prominent visual hallucinations, which get worse over time. Therapy psychiatrists (at least the few who will treat patients with grubby physical illnesses) have developed a brilliant psychotherapeutic approach for these patients. The patient is told to sit up straight in a straight-backed chair. (The couch in this instance must not be utilized). Then, in order to determine if the patient is a candidate for deep psychoanalytic psychotherapy encompassing brilliant, concise interpretations over at least two years, the therapy psychiatrist sits directly in front of the hallucinating patient and makes firm eye contact. Then the psychiatrist voices the following clearly at least three times: "You do not need to hallucinate. This is your opportunity to snap out of it. It is bad for your self-esteem to allow this shameful business to continue. At the count of three you will stop. One … two … three."

If the patient does not stop, refer directly back to the neurologist.

Expertise in treating Parkinson's disease psychosis is critical. It occurs in a few select locations at specialty medical schools, involving close collaboration between the neurologist and brain psychiatrist. (Again, forget most of the country!)

The illness is relatively common. There are characteristic visual hallucinations of which the patient is aware, which slowly worsen. There are a number of potential causes. The treatment for PD with dopaminergic medications most likely plays a role in precipitating hallucinations, so it is a fine line between too much, just enough, and too little. Expertise is required to make these subtle adjustments.

The complex pathophysiology of PD increases vulnerability to

---

[102] "Pathophysiology and Treatment of Psychosis in Parkinson's Disease: a review." Zahodne, B., etc.) *Drugs and Aging.* 2008; 25(8): 665–82.

psychosis, including visual-processing deficits, neurotransmitter abnormalities (dopamine, serotonin, acetylcholine, etc.), structural brain abnormalities involving deposition of Lewy bodies in certain brain areas, and abnormal genetics (for apolipoprotein E, epsilon 4 allele, and tau protein H1H1).

The treatments of choice, once the dopaminergic drug is lowered as much as possible, are antipsychotics. A particular drug, clozapine, has particular efficacy, but it requires expert prescribing and laboratory monitoring. Quetiapine has not been determined to be of benefit in two randomized controlled trials, but because it seemed to help in less definitive (open-label) trials, it is considered the antipsychotic of choice because of its tolerability and relatively benign side effect profile.

A recent double-blind, placebo-controlled trial that enrolled 188 PD patients with hallucinations supported the efficacy of rivastigmine, a cholinesterase inhibitor. Electroconvulsive therapy can be helpful in patients with accompanying depression, suicidality, or refractoriness to treatment with medications. There is also preliminary evidence that two antidepressants, clomipramine (a tricyclic) or citalopram (a serotonergic SSRI), may help a few patients.

Multiple Sclerosis

Multiple sclerosis is a debilitating disease and the leading cause of nontraumatic neurological disability in young people. The etiology is unknown. It can result in a wide variety of neurological symptoms, visual disturbances, dystonia of muscles, and emotional abnormalities. In some cases, there is progressive deterioration of neurological function, particularly paresis of musculature. Other cases have episodic symptoms and don't progress as swiftly. Others may have an even better outcome, a milder remitting-relapsing form that may progress very slowly. Many MS patients end up in wheelchairs and need assistance with ADLs. Well, shouldn't anybody with MS become very depressed? Aren't they all very depressed? Wouldn't you be?

The title of the following article speaks for itself: "Depression in multiple sclerosis: a review."[103] Patients with multiple sclerosis have a particularly high prevalence of depression: 25 percent are clinically depressed in any given year, and 50 percent are clinically depressed over the life span. The prevalence for depression in MS is high even when compared with patients with other chronic illnesses, yet MS patients are rarely screened or treated for depression. This is in spite of a suicide rate of 5 percent. MS patients with depression may have additional brain lesions (added to lesions due to MS alone), more hyperintense lesions in the left interior medial frontal regions, and greater atrophy of the left anterior temporal parietal regions. The proportion of suicides as a cause of death is 7.5 times greater than for an age-matched general population.

A study by Feinstein examined 140 consecutive patients attending an MS clinic in Canada. He reported a lifetime prevalence for suicidal intent of 28.6 percent; of forty patients, nine (6.4 percent) had suicide attempts. Of particular concern from that study was "two-thirds of these patients with current major depression were not receiving antidepressants or any psychological assistance."

Depression in MS increases cognitive impairment: 46 percent have cognitive impairment, 34 percent have memory problems, and 33 percent have executive problems. The degree and pattern of cognitive impairment correlated with disease of white matter tracts within the cerebral hemispheres. Symptoms of depression, apathy, lack of interest, irritability, hopelessness, and suicidal ruminations add to the total disease burden and suffering of MS patients. The authors wrote, "Perhaps the important message here for clinicians is that screening for depression and monitoring of mood should be a feature of the medical management of all patients with MS."

The authors mention that untreated depression is likely to worsen. Depression in MS can be treated, often responding to antidepressants skillfully prescribed and/or a specific form of cognitive therapy

---

[103] Sieger R. J., Abernethy, D. A. "Depression in Multiple Sclerosis: A Review." *Jl. Neurol Neurosurg Psychiatry* 2005; 76 469–475.

emphasizing acquiring coping skills. The authors conclude: "The outstanding question continues to be why depression in people with MS is so infrequently treated?"

The authors couldn't possibly know the reason. The reason is the treachery of the treacherous dichotomy. As long as therapy psychiatry defines depression as a mental health problem in *The Diagnostic and Statistical Manual of Mental Disorders*, it will be trivialized, stigmatized, and ignored!

If it is too much of burden for neurologists or primary care practitioners to screen for depression utilizing brief rating scales like the BDI or HAM-D, a professor, R. L. Spitzer, MD, at Columbia Presbyterian Medical School has developed an extremely brief method, a screen with merely two questions, which rules out or rules in depression with great accuracy.[104]

1. During the past month, have you often been bothered by feeling down or depressed?
2. During the past month, have you often been bothered by having little interest or pleasure in activities you previously enjoyed?

There! It will take five seconds to ask question 1 and an additional five seconds to follow up with the second question. (Is that too much of a burden to save a life or reduce suffering?) This two-questions instrument is 96 percent sensitive in identifying depression if yes is the answer to both, and only 2 percent of individuals who reply no to both will have depression.

That is when the physician should have a brain psychiatrist to refer to expeditiously. The brain psychiatrist must understand neurological illnesses and their treatments, be aware of possible drug interactions when psychiatric drugs must be added to neurological medications, and understand psychiatric diagnosis because patients with

[104] "Recommendation on Diagnosis and Treatment of Depression in Patients with Multiple Sclerosis." Fragoso, Y. D., et al. *Pract Neurol.* 2014: 14(4): 206–209.

neurological illnesses can have a spectrum of psychiatric disorders: bipolar disorder, OCD, panic disorder, other anxiety disorders, and varieties of alcohol and substance abuse. He should also understand the brain pathologies of depression when added to those of MS.

HPV

How can a mental health problem possibly have any influence on a virus? After all, viruses—though minute in size—are real physical entities. HPV that lingers in a woman's body eventually can lead to cervical cancer. New research[105] has linked stress and depression, and the two are often in an intimate linkage to the persistence of the human papillomavirus (HPV) in women.

"Psychosocial Stress, Maladaptive Coping, and HPV Persistence" monitored 333 young women over an eleven-year period starting when they were nineteen. They were evaluated every six months, and at the end of the study, completed a questionnaire that asked about the degree of stress they had and if they were depressed. In a proportion of women, the infection had cleared, and in others, it persisted over the ten-year period.

In general, the virus is cleared in about two years. Anna-Barbara Moscicki, MD, FAAP, chief of the Division of Adolescent and Young Adult Medicine at the University of California School of Medicine found that women who were depressed or perceived themselves to have lots of stress were more likely to have HPV persistence then those with who reported self-destructive coping strategies, like drinking, smoking, cigarettes or taking drugs when stressed. (Of course, unrecognized and untreated depression increases the likelihood of such behaviors). Since the means of reporting depression was a self-reporting questionnaire, it is unclear how many of the stressed and self-destructive subjects were actually clinically depressed.

Dr. Moscicki explained how previous studies have shown stress

---

105 From the Pediatric Academic Societies Meeting, April 30–May 3, 2016, Baltimore, Maryland.

can lead to a greater numbers of herpes virus attacks (in those infected with that virus) and worse medical outcomes for cancer. She summarized, "HPV infections are the cause of cervical cancers. But HPV infections are extremely common, and only the few infections that continue years beyond initial infection are at risk of developing cervical cancer." She added, "This is alarming since many of these women acquired their persistent infection as adolescents."

It is a safe bet that the role of depression was not seriously addressed and remained untreated. After all, it's merely a mental health problem, according to the specialty of psychiatry.

Comorbid Pain

By middle age, nearly everybody has experienced some form of real physical pain, which unlike mental pain is evoked by dysfunction in some part of the real physical body. People with mental problems should be grateful they do not have real physical pain, which really does hurt! Many therapy psychiatrists believe attacking even physical pain with brilliant, targeted, incisive interpretations, aimed at deeply buried conflicts in the id and superego, will alleviate it, as psychodynamic psychotherapy over two or more years does for mental pain. Of course, mental pain, because it is of such a lesser degree than physical pain, actually may not need alleviation, so why is two or three years of psychodynamic psychotherapy necessary to begin with?

Think back to the last time you had real physical pain. Was it a severe toothache? A fractured bone in a limb? Severe stomach distress with nausea and vomiting? Or getting punched very hard in the face? That's pain—real physical pain. How can so-called mental pain even compare in magnitude and suffering experienced? Real physical pain has its origins in the obvious damage to actual physical organs in contrast to the mere emotions associated with mental pain.

There are several candidate genes for chronic pain.[106] One of the

---

[106] Ramezani, A, PhD, et al., chronic pain and psychiatric illness, managing comorbid conditions. *Current Psychiatry* February 2016, 15(2): 26.33

most studied is 5-HTTLPR, which is involved in regulating synthesis of the serotonin transporter (a reuptake pump) that brings serotonin back into the neuron. Both monoamines and inflammatory cytokines play a role in modulating gamma-aminobutyric acid (GABA) and glutamate neurons as well as glial cells constituting peripheral pain pathways and central circuits that participate in the pain response.

Particular genes associated with pain are those regulating serotonin 5-HT2A and 5-HT1A receptors, catechol-o methyltransferase (an enzyme involved in catechol metabolism), the dopamine D4 receptor, and pro-inflammatory cytokines, interleukin-1 and interleukin-6. Particular brain circuitry is involved in processing pain stimuli, referred to as the pain matrix, which is a complex aggregate of interconnected brain structures involved in evoking defensive responses to pain.

Imaging studies show that the dorsal anterior cingulate mediates distress in response to pain. Emerging structural imaging provides evidence of continuous reorganization of prefrontal cortices. Of particular interest[107] are findings of a reduction of gray matter in the dorsolateral prefrontal cortex (DLPFC), given that it is a hub of the cognitive and executive function deficits. Likewise, the mPFC (medial-prefrontal cortex) is a key component of the default mode network (DMN), a functional network also comprising the posterior cingulate cortex and hippocampus.

Negative neuroplastic changes in the DMN are a common finding in chronic pain. Functional and structural changes in the amygdala and hippocampus have been described in fibromyalgia and neuropathic pain. Dysfunction in these limbic formations may be a contributing factor in the disruption of neuroendocrine and autonomic and immune function, which could further contribute to pain symptoms. Consequently, excessive hypothalamic-pituitary-adrenal axis and sympathetic activation combined with elevation of

---

[107] Maletic V., MD, MS, DeMuri, Bernadette, MD, "Chronic Pain and Depression: Understanding 2 Culprits in Common." *Current Psychiatry*, February 2016, 15(2) 40–44, 52, 54.

proinflammatory cytokine production, and release likely plays a role in the pathophysiology of pain. Pain is associated with perturbed neuron-glia relationships, altered glutamatergic, GABA, glycine, substance-P, opioid, 5-HT, norepinephrine and dopamine signaling, dysfunction of intracellular signaling cascades, and neuropathic signaling.

Pain disorders are associated with an estimated annual cost of $600 billion, not counting lost time from employment and other responsibilities.[108] Pain can be categorized as *neuropathic* or *nociceptive*. Neuropathic pain can be described by patients as numbness, burning, electric-like, and tingling, and it results from damage to nerves. Nociceptive pain is represented by toothaches, acute injuries, or trauma and is described as sharp or stabbing or as a dull, aching pain. Nociceptive pain is treated with anti-inflammatory drugs like NSAIDS, acetaminophen, and nonselective COX inhibitors (ibuprofen, indomethacin). Neuropathic pain is treated with certain antidepressants that are dual agents, increasing serotonin and norepinephrine (tricyclic antidepressants) or SNRIs like duloxetine or venlafaxine.

The other group of medications with efficacy in treating neuropathic pain are anticonvulsants (gabapentin and pregabalin are the most frequently used). The prescription of opioid pain medication is associated with higher risk of adverse reactions or complications, and patients should be carefully selected if they are prescribed. Inclusion of cognitive-behavioral therapy and other interventional procedures such as physical therapy are employed.

One need not be a genius to realize mental pain as a symptom of MDD—and not caused by physical damage to nerves or body tissue. It does not have a significant underlying physical basis. Therapy psychiatrists, as mentioned previously, are strongly inclined to uproot mental pain by digging out the deep psychological conflicts that cause it in the process of deep psychoanalytic psychotherapy. However,

---

[108] Ramezani, A, PD, et al, "Chronic pain and psychiatric illness managing comorbid conditions," *Current Psychiatry* 2016, February; 15(2): 26–33.

some brave souls, usually neurologists, neuropathologists, and even some brain psychiatrists decided to buck that trend to ascertain if in MDD there could be underlying biological dysregulations, causing symptoms in a fashion similar to physical pain. Some therapy psychiatrists learning of this work were openly skeptical that this would be a fatuous endeavor and a waste of research funds.

Nevertheless, the researchers over the past ten plus years have plowed ahead, and even though the therapy psychiatrists have discredited their research, the following are the general findings:

There are several candidate genes for major depressive disorder. One of the most studied is 5-HTTLPR, which is involved in regulating synthesis of the serotonin transporter (a reuptake pump) that brings serotonin back into the neuron. Both monoamines and inflammatory cytokines play a role in modulating gamma-aminobutyric acid (GABA) and glutamate neurons as well as glial cells, constituting peripheral mood-regulating pathways and central circuits that participate in producing the symptoms of MDD.

Particular genes associated with MDD are those regulating serotonin 5-HT2A and 5-HT1A receptors, catechol-O-methyltransferase (an enzyme involved in catechol metabolism), the dopamine D4 receptor, and proinflammatory cytokines interleukin-1 and interleukin-6. Imaging studies show that the dorsal anterior cingulate mediates distress in response to emotional pain. Emerging structural imaging provides evidence of continuous reorganization of the prefrontal cortex.

Of particular interest are findings of a reduction of gray matter in the dorsolateral prefrontal cortex (DLPFC), given that it is a hub of the so-called cognitive and executive function deficits. Likewise, the MPFC is a key component of the default mode network (DMN), a functional network also comprising the posterior cingulate cortex and hippocampus. Negative neuroplastic change in the DMN are a common finding in MDD. Functional and structural changes in the amygdala and hippocampus have been described in MDD. Dysfunction in these limbic formations may be a contributing factor in the disruption of neuroendocrine, autonomic, and immune function, which could further contribute to symptoms of MDD. Consequently, excessive hypothalamic-pituitary-adrenal axis and sympathetic activation combined with elevation of pro-inflammatory cytokine production and release likely play a role in the pathophysiology of MDD. MDD is associated with perturbed neuron-glial relationships, altered glutamatergic, GABA, glycine substance-P1 opioid, 5-HT, norepinephrine and dopamine signaling, dysfunction of intracellular signaling cascades, and neuropathic signaling.[109]

Maybe MDD is not a mental health problem after all and should be taken as seriously as chronic pain disorders (which nobody is claiming are mental problems). The pathological (physical) brain mechanisms underlying both seem equally physical, and parallel each other to a very close degree.

Substance Abuse

There is an extremely high comorbidity between alcohol and drug use disorder and other mental illnesses.[110] Diagnosis of a mental illness may not occur until the symptoms have caused gross disruptions in the patient's life or family routines or serious manifestations in public, academic, vocational, or social settings. The symptoms in milder form may have been present for years—neither diagnosed nor treated until a crisis level is reached. In order to obtain relief from these milder or prodromal symptoms, individuals may turn to alcohol, cannabis, or harder drugs, and in many instances, they will obtain momentary relief. But because these are addictive substances, many individuals will progress to outright addiction, creating a dual-diagnosis syndrome, a full-blown addiction, and an exacerbated mental illness, usually leaving the ailing individual's life in utter shambles. Unless

---

[109] Maletic, MS, Valentino, MOD, MS, DeMuri, Bernadette, MOD: "Chronic Pain and Depression: Understanding 2 Culprits in Common," *Current Psychiatry*, February 2016, 15(2) 40–44, 52, 54.

[110] "Comorbidity: Addiction and Other Mental Illnesses," National institute of Mental Health.

a powerful therapeutic intervention is available, these individuals' lives can be written off as far as contributing to society, insidiously sinking into a pit of profound mental and physical illness, disability, and premature death. For family members, there is the concomitant hell of helplessly watching their loved one turn into a vegetable.

SAMHSA (Substance Abuse and Mental Health Services Administration) has presented a paper called "Mental and Substance Use Disorders." In the overview section, they point out that these illnesses affect people from all walks of life and all age groups. According to the 2014 National Survey on Drug Use and Health, an estimated 43.6 million people (18.1 percent of Americans ages eighteen and up experience some form of mental illness. Over a year period, 20.2 million adults (8.4 percent) had a substance abuse disorder. Of these, 7.9 million people had a dual diagnosis, both a mental illness and substance abuse.

Serious Mental Illness

Serious mental illness among people ages eighteen and older is defined at the federal level as having, at any time during the past year, a diagnosable mental, behavioral, or emotional disorder that causes serious functional impairment that substantially interferes with or limits one or more major life activities. Serious mental illnesses include major depression, schizophrenia, bipolar disorder, and other mental disorders that cause serious impairment. In 2014, an estimated 9.8 million adults (4.1 percent) ages eighteen and up had suffered a serious mental illness in the past year. People with serious mental illness are more likely to be unemployed, arrested, and/or face inadequate housing compared to those without mental illness.

Serious Emotional Disturbance

The term *serious emotional disturbance* (SED) is used to refer to children and youth who have had a diagnosable mental, behavioral, or emotional disorder in the past year, which resulted in functional impairment that substantially interfered with or limited the child's role or function in family, school, or community activities. A Centers for Disease Control and Prevention (CDC) review of population-level information found that estimates of the number of children with a mental disorder range from 13–20 percent, but current national surveys do not have an indicator of SED.

Substance Use Disorders

Substance use disorders occur when the recurrent use of alcohol and/or drugs causes clinically significant impairment, including health problems, disability, and failure to meet major responsibilities at work, school, or home.

In 2014, about 21.5 million Americans ages twelve and older (8.1 percent) were classified with a substance use disorder in the past year. Of those, 2.6 million had problems with both alcohol and drugs, 4.5 million had problems with drugs but not alcohol, and 14.4 million had problems with alcohol only.

Co-occurring Mental and Substance Use Disorders

The coexistence of both a mental health and a substance use disorder is referred to as *co-occurring disorders*. According to SAMHSA's 2014 National Survey on Drug Use and Health, approximately 7.9 million adults had co-occurring disorders in 2014. During the past year, for those adults surveyed who experienced substance use disorders and mental illness, rates were highest among adults ages twenty-six to forty-nine (42.7 percent). For adults with past-year serious mental illness and co-occurring substance use disorders, rates were highest among those ages eighteen to twenty-five (35.3 percent) in 2014.

GLOSSARY

agonist. A chemical that, when binding to a receptor, produces a biological response.

allelic variants. A gene can have a number of alternative forms. Generally, they result in little or no observable variation in traits they code for.

antagonist. A chemical that, when binding to a receptor, turns off the biological response.

anterior and posterior cingulate. Part of limbic cortex. It includes the cingulate gyrus, receives input from the thalamus and neocortex, and is involved in emotion formation and processing.

augmentation strategy. The addition of another drug or other drugs to boost the efficacy of the original drug.

basal ganglia. They comprise multiple subcortical nuclei. (A nucleus is a dense concentration of neurons in a particular location). They are strongly interconnected with the cerebral cortex, thalamus, and brain stem. They are associated with a variety of functions including control of voluntary motor movements, procedural learning, routine behavior or habits, eye movements, cognition, and emotion.

cingulate: (anterior, posterior, subcallosal). A part of the limbic system, with subsections playing a role in cognition.

copy number variants. Chromosome modifications may arise during normal cell processes and, if left unrepaired, may cause chromosome damage, which can result in genetic changes.

deep-brain stimulation. A neurosurgical procedure involving the implanting of a medical device termed a neurostimulator, which sends electrical impulses through implanted electrodes. It can provide benefits for Parkinson's disease, chronic pain, MDD, and OCD.

endogenous neurotransmitter. They are supplied by the brain itself, and include serotonin, dopamine, norepinephrine, and a multiplicity of others.

epistatic effects (of genes). When one gene is dependent on the presence of a modifier gene for expression, it can result in a double mutation.

frontal cortex, medial. Part of the frontal lobe, which plays a role in decision-making and possibly slow-wave sleep.

frontal gyrus, superior. Makes up about one-third of the frontal lobes and contributes to higher cognitive functions, especially working memory.

glutamatergic A1 and A2 receptors. The neurotransmitter glutamate binds to them. Glutamate is an excitatory neurotransmitter, which if excessive, can damage axons and dendrites and even cause apoptosis (when a neuron destroys itself according to a built-in suicide mechanism).

hypometabolic. A state of reduced metabolism that can result in a wide variety of dysfunctions in the brain.

insula. A portion of the cerebral cortex involved in emotional processing. It is folded deep into the lateral sulcus, the fissure separating the temporal from the parietal lobe.

internal capsule. A white matter structure deeply located in the brain. It is composed of axons from the motor cortex on their way to muscles. Damage can result in paralysis. It is situated in each cerebral hemisphere, passing by the basal ganglia and separating the caudate nucleus and thalamus from the putamen and globus pallidus.

lateral dorsal prefrontal cortex. An area of the prefrontal cortex. Primary functions include decision-making, working memory, and social cognition. It has clinical significance in schizophrenia, depression, stress, and alcohol and substance abuse.

lateral and medial temporal cortex. The temporal cortex is one of the four major lobes of the brain and is particularly important for declarative and long-term memory.

MAOI antidepressant. A subtype of antidepressant requiring a prescriber who has special proficiency in its prescription. It may be efficacious if other antidepressants have failed, but it can have serious side effects if not monitored properly.

medial forebrain bundle. A white matter tract containing fibers from the olfactory regions considered to be part of the reward system for pleasure. It can be targeted in the treatment of severe depression (MDD) with deep-brain stimulation treatment.

medial/frontal cortex (mPFC). Plays important roles in decision-making, error detection, executive control, and decision-making about risk and reward of a behavior.

NMDAr (receptor). A glutamate receptor. It is very important in controlling synaptic plasticity and memory function. Hypofunction is associated with learning impairments, memory impairments, and under certain conditions, psychosis.

nucleus accumbens. A major component of the reward system. It is considered part of the basal ganglia and the main component of the ventral striatum.

occipital cortex. One of the four major lobes of the cerebral cortex. It serves as the visual processing center.

plasticity. Said of any working element of a neuron, axons, dendrites, synapses, and networks. The greater the plasticity, the more optimal the functioning.

prefrontal cortex, left dorsal. An area of the prefrontal cortex involved in working memory tasks.

receptors, glutamatergic A1 and A2. Subtypes of receptors that bind glutamate, an excitatory neurotransmitter.

sensorimotor areas. Combining the motor area of the cortex, which plans and executes movement, with the five sensory systems of the brain. They are anatomically distinct, but they can work in synchrony.

subcallosal cingulate gyrus. A portion of the cingulum that is an important node in a network that includes cortical structures, the limbic system, thalamus, hypothalamus, and brain stem nuclei.

There is abnormal metabolic activity in depression that may serve as a therapeutic target for deep-brain stimulation treatment.

temporal cortex, lateral and medial. The medial temporal cortex is vital for long-term memory.

tricyclic antidepressants. An older type of antidepressant that may have efficacy in case newer varieties don't. The prescriber must have experience with laboratory measurements and electrocardiograms.

vagus nerve. The tenth cranial nerve supplies parasympathetic innervations to the heart, lungs, and digestive tract. In contrast to sympathetic innervations, it slows the heart. It can play a role in the treatment of MDD.

ventral capsule/striatum. A major portion of the basal ganglia that functions as part of the reward system. It has been a target for treatment of MDD using deep-brain stimulation.

visual areas. Visual cortex in the region of the occipital cortex. Integrates all input into a comprehensive picture.

CHAPTER 22

Do You Still Believe?

It would seem counterintuitive to compare the relative sufferings and disabilities of people afflicted with mental health issue to those having to contend with real physical medical diseases. Why write a lengthy narrative on such a topic when common sense alone should dictate the latter are really physical, disrupting, impairing, even destroying real bodily tissue, while the former are the ethereal products of the mind, thoughts, emotions, and complaints!

The World Health Organization[111] reports an estimated 350 million people are affected by depression, and 800,000 die by suicide each year. By depression, they do not mean reactive mood changes due to adversity, but persistent symptoms, depressed mood, loss of the capacity to maintain interest or enjoy previously enjoyable activities (anhedonia), reduced energy and levels of activity, disturbed sleep and appetite, feelings of guilt and low self-worth, impaired concentration, anxiety, hopelessness, and suicidality. They note the relationship between depression and physical health—depression and worsening of cardiovascular disease and vice versa—as well as impairments in the capacity to function in core life roles at work, at school, and at home. In underdeveloped countries, fewer than 10 percent get any help, and even in developed countries, it is less than 50 percent. (This

[111] World Health Organization, Media Centre, "Depression Fact Sheet." Reviewed April 2016.

author has commented on the gross unevenness of the quality of that help in the United States).

Jean-Pierre Lepine and Mike Briley wrote "The Increasing Burden of Depression."[112] They report depression is among the leading causes of burden of diseases worldwide. The World Health Organization projects it will be the leading cause of disease burden by 2030, outpacing all the so-called physical illnesses like cardiovascular disease and cancer.

All studies of depression stress it results in increased disease burden from other illnesses, high levels of disability, and significantly higher mortality from all causes in comparison to individuals without depression. It magnifies the risk of developing cardiovascular diseases and stroke, and it worsens the prognosis.

In a study of 896 patients hospitalized for myocardial infarction (heart attack), it increased the risk of death in those who had depression. A meta-analysis of twenty studies found depression doubled the risk of death for heart patients in the next three to six months, and by two years, the rate had increased more than two and a half times.

Another study measured long-term mortality rates in 12,866 men with a high risk of coronary artery disease. Those who also had depression had double the risk of death. In another study from Australia, 883 men were followed for six years. Those with the most severe depressions had a 3.32 higher risk of dying! Suicide is not the main cause of death in the clinically depressed, even though the suicide rate is twenty times greater for men, and twenty-seven times greater for women than in the general population.

The burden of depression doesn't just apply to those who die directly or indirectly from it, but also the degradation of the abilities, functioning, and quality of life of those who suffer from it. Work ability falls off, resulting in poorer performance, absenteeism, and unemployment. The concomitant loss of income stresses the patient and the family. There is a rise in separations and divorces, and even in families that remain intact, there is a financial squeeze. Depressed

---

[112] "Neuropsychiatric Disease Treatment 2011," 7 (Suppl 1): 3–7.

mothers may not be able to emotionally support their children with psychological and developmental consequences. The authors quote a statistic from the National Comorbidity Survey Replication, a US nationally representative household survey, that overall impairment was significantly higher for mental disorders (42 percent of persons) than for physical (24 percent). In spite of these facts, according to their statistics, only 21.4 percent of those with mental disorders receive treatment in contrast to 58.2 percent with medical disorders. And they comment that the treatments often are not fully effective. Most patients still have residual symptoms, especially cognitive impairment or social dysfunction, and reduced performance capacities, resulting in ongoing distress. And the risk of relapse weighs on them: 60 percent in five years, 67 percent in ten years, and 85 percent after fifteen years.

It should be clear that depression is a burdensome disease and not just a mental health problem. One has to constantly fight the pervasive ignorance extant in society perpetuated by therapy-psychiatry, which results in the trivialization, minimization, and stigmatization of depression. Psychiatry is averse to really destigmatizing mental illness even though they glibly state they are against the stigma, but as long as depression is defined as mental, that is how long the stigma will be perpetuated. And they have a powerful incentive to keep it mental so they can continue psychodynamic psychotherapy forty-five-minute talk sessions once or more times a week for several years with each patient, yielding a nice income stream. I guess one can't blame them since many are trapped by that income stream.

However, there are purely physical treatments for depression in the same manner as for neurological and medical illnesses. Of course, pharmacology, provided by experienced physicians, is the predominant mode of treatment in all medical specialties; even surgical specialties utilize it adjunctively. Neurology, the other medical specialty focusing on the brain and its functions, has a large array of medications to treat neurological diseases.

It is the mental business that influences the mind-set of the therapy psychiatrists and a host of non-MD therapists (who cannot prescribe), the media, and much of the public, which insists mental illness is different because it's not of the stuff of the brain. Everybody has an opinion on mental illness! Pharmacology is just as important in treating mental illnesses as epilepsy or heart disease. It is now a full-fledged medical specialty like any other, using combinations of medications to alleviate symptoms—if the prescriber is a brain psychiatrist-clinical psychopharmacologist.

Pharmacology is a purely physical treatment. (One not need know at all about the deep psychological conflicts in the id and the superego). However, there are additional, purely physical treatments for the mental health problems in *The Diagnostic and Statistical Manual of Mental Disorders.* My heavens! Symptoms that respond to purely physical treatments might not be mental symptoms at all. Indeed, if mental illnesses really aren't mental illnesses, that has revolutionary implications. All psychiatrists should rip up their mental manual once and for all. It never hurts to review the physical causes of psychiatric disorders because our individual and collective minds have been bombarded with a century of propaganda that they are categorically mental health problems.

Before going into detail about the roster of purely physical treatments, it is helpful to be more informed about neuroimaging of the brain. By now, hundreds of thousands of brain scans have been taken on a similar number of patients. To date, there has only been one instance when a therapy psychiatrist somehow found himself in the radiology department of a community hospital and viewed a scan. He was certain he had identified both the id and the superego in the scan of one of his patients. Apart from that exception, no neurologist or radiologist has been able to confirm that therapy psychiatrist's findings in any brain scan. (Of course, they probably were not really looking for the id or the superego).

A massive scientific study was completed in Great Britain.[113] It is

---

[113] "Neuroimaging distinction between neurological and psychiatric disorders," Crossley N., Scott J., Ellison-Wright, I., and Mechelli, A. *The British Journal of Psychiatry*, Nov. 2015, 207 (5) 429–434.

fortunate the study was conducted and completed there since there are proportionally far fewer therapy psychiatrists to muddle the research or protest its findings. According to the authors of the article, over the past few years, the distinction between psychiatric and neurological disorders has been called into question on the latest scientific data. Neurological disorders can present with affective (mood) symptoms and psychotic symptoms, and psychiatric disorders can present with motor (physical) neurological symptoms. They consider the view of therapy psychiatrists that neurological disorders are "organic" (physical), and psychiatric disorders are functional (mental).

It's no surprise that therapy psychiatrists hold simplistic notions about the etiologies and causes of their favorite category of illness: mental illness.

The authors show how the neuroscientific evidence and genetic studies have begun to reveal the biological underpinnings of both neurological and psychiatric disorders. Such data include all allelic variants, copy number variants, and epistatic effects, and gene-environment interactions play a critical role in both sets of disorders.

Brave researchers have tried to end the distinction between mental and neurological illnesses.[114] If White had made this comment in the United States, thirty thousand therapy psychiatrists would have lynched him!

Emerging scientific evidence suggests the presence of comparable etiological mechanisms and that the current distinction between disorders of the mind and disorders of the brain is a fundamental misconception that calls for a radical rethinking in which psychiatric disorders should be reclassified as disorders of the central nervous system—including the brain! That would be entirely logical since neurological and psychiatric disorders are rooted in the brain.

This author has wondered, by playing a part in transforming mental illness into physical diseases of the brain and central nervous system, if a wild-eyed therapy psychiatrist will plot some revenge.

---

[114] (White, P. D., Rickards, H., Zeman A. Z., "Time to end the distinction between mental and neurological illnesses. *BMJ*, 2012; 344.)

When this book is published, I have no doubt a cacophony of Sturm und Drang from therapy psychiatrists will follow!

The authors state any new classification must be informed by scientific evidence, including the biology underpinning the two classes of disorders. Their study investigated whether neurological and psychiatric disorders have distinct neuroimaging correlates, whether the two classes of disorders affected different sets of brain regions, whether these regions were localized in different functional networks, and whether neuroanatomical variability within each class of disorders is smaller than between classes. Their research was based on meta-analysis of 168 published scientific studies involving a total of 4,227 patients and matched 4,504 healthy controls. The results of the study found both types of disorders were associated with widespread alterations in cortical and subcortical brain areas.

Therapy psychiatrists generally avoid reading the neuroscientific literature, so it is unlikely any read the conclusions stated in this article. This is fortunate since huge amounts of anti-ulcer medications would have been required to sooth their gastro symptoms. Of course, an alternative to anti-ulcer medication could be two or more years of psychoanalytically oriented psychotherapy, but then every therapy psychiatrist in the country would be tied up treating other therapy psychiatrists.

The results of the study demonstrated that there are many biological similarities between the two sets of disorders, and this similarity is driven by the network organization of the brain, which provides fresh support for a new conceptual framework in which neurological and psychiatric disorders are both considered disorders of the nervous system. Although there were many similar brain regions affected by both types of disorders, their meta-analytic techniques also showed differences between the two groups. The basal ganglia, insula, lateral and medial temporal cortex, and sensorimotor motor areas showed greater impairment in neurological disorders, whereas the medial frontal cortex, anterior and posterior cingulate, superior frontal gyrus, and occipital cortex (bilateral lingual gyrus and left cuneus) showed greater impairment in psychiatric disorders. Those structural differences between the two classes of disorders affected distinct functional networks. The psychiatric disorders had a greater effect in visual areas than the neurological disorders. So, in summary, both neurological and psychiatric disorders have many *biological* abnormalities in common, but they also have some distinct differences.

Purely Physical Treatment: Deep-Brain Stimulation

The Mayo Clinic in Minnesota was recognized as the best neurology and neurosurgery hospital in the nation for 2015–2016 by *US News and World Report*. Deep-brain stimulation is used to treat a number of neurological conditions (which are real physical illnesses or symptoms) such as severe tremor, Parkinson's disease, epilepsy, dystonia, Tourette's syndrome, and chronic pain for which medications have failed to satisfactorily alleviate symptoms. This procedure involves surgery, during which the surgeon implants a thin wire lead into specific areas of the brain. The implanted wire is threaded under the skin to a pulse generator (neurostimulator) implanted near the collarbone. The generator is then programmed to send electrical pulses to the brain. The degree and timing of the stimulation are regulated by the physician and customized for the particular symptoms requiring control.

Therapy psychiatrists do acknowledge deep-brain stimulation may help neurological diseases and symptoms, but they refute such a primitive physical treatment could possibly be of use in mental illness, in which complex deeply buried unconscious conflicts are structurally interwoven in the id and superego. No simple wire implanted in the brain can induce anything more than the most superficial, transitory relief of symptoms.

Nevertheless, some proactive physicians, willing to brave the derision and contempt of the therapy psychiatrists, have used this grubby, simplistic, physical treatment to treat MDD and OCD. Even the Mayo Clinic has braved the contempt of the therapy psychiatrists by offering deep-brain stimulation for the treatment of MDD and OCD.

What? Using this purely physical treatment for a mental health problem? Well, at the Mayo Clinic, they must know what they're doing!

The results of an original scientific study of DBS in MDD was published April 6, 2016.[115] Treatment-resistant depression (TRD) is defined by the failure of systematic usual treatment, i.e. four unsuccessful trials on antidepressants and failure to respond to ECT. TRD is associated with more hospitalizations, more suicide attempts, and higher costs compared to non-TRD patients. Twenty-five TRD patients in the Netherlands were selected for a scientific study termed a randomized, double-blind, twelve-week phase with a subsequent twelve-week crossover phase. Thus, for twelve weeks, half received DBS and half sham DBS, and then the DBS versus sham was reversed. The electrode wires were inserted into a specific brain area: the ventral anterior limb of the internal capsule. At the end of the study, ten patients were classified as responders (40 percent), and an additional six patients (24 percent) were classified as partial responders. Of the responders, five (20 percent) had a complete alleviation of symptoms or remission.

For the 30 percent of patients who fail more routine treatments, DBS may offer hope. The technique is underactive exploration, particularly in the selection of different sites in the brain involved in the neurobiology of MDD: the subcallosal cingulate gyrus, the medial forebrain bundle, the ventral capsule/ventral-striatum, and the nucleus accumbens. The procedure appears safe and has few adverse effects.

Therapy psychiatrists have put names to many psychological defenses, mental mechanisms to avoid emotional pain, or prevent painful conflicts from entering awareness. Two similar defenses are

---

[115] Bergfeld, Isidoor MSc et al., "Deep-Brain Stimulation of the Ventral Anterior Limb of the Internal Capsule for Treatment-Resistant Depression," *JAMA Psychiatry*. Published online April 6, 2016.

suppression (the individual is aware of the painful circumstance but pushes it out of consciousness to ignore it) or repression (keeping a painful conflict or emotion deeply buried in the unconscious).

Can a grubby neurosurgical procedure like DBS actually benefit mental health problems? Suppression and repression are both highly prevalent among therapy psychiatrists.

Another purely physical treatment for therapy psychiatrists to suppress or repress transcranial magnetic stimulation of MDD. TMS is used to treat severe migraine and tinnitus, which are real physical symptoms. However, some enterprising physicians and researchers thought they'd give it a shot with mental health problems. How could it be? It turned out this simple purely physical, grubby treatment can be beneficial for the mental cases with depression, obsessive-compulsive disorder, posttraumatic stress disorder, and schizophrenia. Oh, wonder of wonders! Many scientifically designed studies have documented TMS efficacy for treating MDD (a total of eighteen that incorporated 1970 patients).

The usual response rate for treatment-resistant depression (TRD) approaches 60 percent (58.0 percent) and has a remission rate of 37.1 percent. The procedure involves a daily treatment with a specially designed magnetic coil placed over the left dorsolateral prefrontal cortex, which has been shown to be hypometabolic in MDD. Blood flow and metabolism in that area of the brain normalize with a course of treatment. The total number of treatment sessions required is twenty to thirty. The procedure is noninvasive, and side effects are infrequent and generally mild. Imaging studies indicate transsynaptic connections with deeper parts of the brain permit beneficial modulation of relevant circuits. After patients respond to acute treatment, because TRD is highly recurrent, maintenance treatments (although much less frequent than acute treatment) are generally scheduled. Researchers are working out the details of maintenance schedules.

Wait! There is still another purely physical treatment that is often effective (and does not require even one deep, incisive interpretation of deep unconscious conflict in the id and superego).

Vagus Nerve Stimulation (VNS)

This procedure has been approved by the FDA for treatment of epilepsy when traditional treatments haven't worked.[116] About 30 percent of epilepsy patients do not respond sufficiently to pharmacological therapy. VNS is added to traditional treatments. Although it's not a cure for epilepsy, it may reduce the frequency of seizures by 50 percent and reduce their intensity. In addition to epilepsy, research is proceeding on its possible benefit for multiple sclerosis, migraines, and Alzheimer's disease (all of which are real physical diseases of the brain!).

VNS requires minor one-day surgery in which a pulse generator is implanted under the skin of the chest and then its connecting wire is threaded under the skin to the left vagus nerve, also in the chest. The left vagus nerve then transmits the impulse up to the brain when it is activated. The physician can regulate the frequency, duration, and intensity of the pulses, and the patient can be taught to self-administer. VNS is not a rapidly working treatment. It can take up to a year and a half for maximum benefit in terms of seizure alleviation to occur.

Thank God for renegades. Some brave physicians were willing to endure the wrath of therapy-psychiatry to learn if this purely physical treatment for neurological illnesses could also be beneficial for mental cases. As for difficult-to-treat neurological disorders, it is reserved for patients with MDD who have responded inadequately to four medication trials and/or ECT. As for neurological disorders, the VNS does not replace the standard treatments. It is used adjunctively; for neurological disorders, the benefits might not be apparent for many months. The FDA has approved VNS for treatment-resistant depression (similarly to epilepsy).

And there's another purely physical treatment that can work in one or two days? (That would leave absolutely no time to dig out those deeply buried conflicts in the id and superego). This fourth purely physical treatment employs a particular molecule, ketamine, rather than a

---

[116] "Vagus Nerve Stimulation," The Mayo Clinic Staff.

device. Ketamine, its metabolites, and numerous other molecules bind to a specific receptor, the N-methyl-D-aspartate receptor (NMDAR).[117] This receptor plays an important role in memory function and learning by promoting optimal functioning of synapses (the connecting nodes between neurons). Its endogenous neurotransmitters are glutamate and glycine. Many exogenous molecules (from outside the body) also modulate it. When a glutaminergic neuron fires, ions of magnesium and zinc, which block the opening, are tossed off so calcium and potassium ions can enter the neuron. Structurally, the NMDAR is quite complex, with a modular design, each module having subunits with different functions. In addition to ketamine, there are at least twenty-nine other molecules with a similar action (antagonism). There are at least eighteen molecules that have the opposite action, agonism, including glutamic acid and the spice curcumin (turmeric).

A case in which the use of ketamine for severe MDD was considered was reviewed in *Current Psychiatry*.[118] The patient, a thirty-one-year-old woman, started having major depressive episodes in her early twenties. She was having at least two per year, lasting eight to ten weeks and interrupting her functioning in her work, her relationships, and her financial security. She underwent at least four antidepressant trials: sertraline (200 mg/day), venlafaxine XR (300 mg/day), bupropion XL (450 mg/day), and vortioxetine (20 mg/day) without relief. A course of ECT did help her mood, but she developed cognitive side effects.

After ECT was terminated, she sought treatment with ketamine. Evidently the consultant informed her there were still several traditional options she should try first, including pharmacological augmentation strategies (thyroid hormone, buspirone, and/or lithium added to her antidepressant) or trials of two alternative classes of antidepressants, tricyclics like desipramine or Nortriptyline, or a trial with an MAO inhibitor like phenelzine or selegiline.)

---

117 "The NMDA Receptor," Wikipedia.

118 "Is the evidence compelling for using ketamine to treat resistant depression?" Nichols, Stephanie, PharmD et al, *Current Psychiatry*, May 2016; 15 (5) 48–51.

This is where expertise comes into play. The consultant, evidently a knowledgeable expert in pharmacology, was aware of several additional traditional treatments that should be utilized *before* going to a more experimental treatment like intravenous ketamine!

Several small studies have utilized ketamine to treat MDD and TRD. A single individual dose is administered, and within twenty-four to forty-eight hours after the infusion, 50–70 percent of patients will show significant improvement in symptoms.

Perhaps the ketamine serves as a solvent in which the deep unconscious conflicts in the id and superego just dissolve rather than requiring two or more years of intensive psychodynamic therapy, which may or may not result in improvement.

Ketamine, in spite of its seeming miraculous efficacy, has a number of problems associated with its use. Often the improvement fades in one or two weeks. There can be adverse effects, including hallucinations and dissociative symptoms, as well as cardiovascular and gastric side effects. If the treatment is repeated, it is not known if tolerance develops to its therapeutic effects. The treatment needs to be administered in a medical center in which anesthesiologists are available. And, of course, ketamine can be a drug of abuse on the street or in the home.

Its experimental nature hasn't stopped private ketamine-infusion centers from setting up shop and claiming very beneficial results with very few serious adverse effects. If one is considering ketamine treatment, it would seem safest to see if it's offered at the best medical school hospitals.

The mechanism of action of ketamine and one specific metabolite are being heavily researched with the hope a new therapeutic armamentarium of rapid-acting antidepressants can be developed.[119] The specific metabolite of ketamine with potential antidepressant action is (2S, 6S, 2R, 6R)-hydroxyl-ketamine, which we'll refer to as HNK. And what a hunk of a molecule it is!

---

[119] "NMDAR inhibition-independent antidepressant actions of ketamine metabolites," Zanos, Panos et al. *Nature* 17998, published online May 4, 2016).

The trick is to obtain the same rapid response without the side effects of ketamine. HNK rapidly increases brain-derived neurotrophic factor (BDNF) in glutamatergic A1 and A2 receptors in the synapses of the mouse hippocampus, which is associated with enhanced synaptic function and an increase in glutamatergic neurotransmission. There is no apparent abuse potential or ketamine-like side effects. Researchers look forward to developing a new generation of rapid-acting antidepressants.

Electroconvulsive Therapy

This purely physical treatment has been around since the 1930s. In *One Flew Over the Cuckoo's Nest,* Jack Nicholson's character received a typical ECT treatment. First, some strong men pinned him to a wall. Another individual applied two paddles, one to each side of the forehead, while Nicholson's character angrily stared at him. The zap was followed by a seizure. The attendants prevented too much flailing about, lowering him to the floor.

Why would any individual submit to such barbarism—no matter how ill they are? Yet 100,000 people receive ECT annually in the United States. Just kidding. ECT is now given in controlled medical settings. The patient is not awake when given the treatment, and the procedure has modified the seizure to such a degree that all that might be apparent during the seizure is slight motion of the toes. After the treatment, the patient is wheeled into the recovery room and attended to by nurses.

ECT is an extremely effective treatment for the most incapacitating severe depressions and/or acute, intense suicidal urges. Usually three treatments are given per week for two to three weeks. It can be given as an outpatient procedure. The most critical factor in the success of ECT are appropriate patient selection, careful monitoring of mood symptoms during the course of ECT to detect improvement response and remission, and ongoing monitoring of the mental status for cognitive or memory side effects. It is a delicate titration.

If the physician ordering the course of ECT is not diligent in those three tasks, the patient may not have a complete response and might become confused or disoriented. In most cases, if the physician is conscientiously monitoring the patient, side effects are few and transitory. Like any complex medical procedure, it is important the physician and the facility are experienced with the treatment.

GLOSSARY

ACC (rostral anterior cingulate cortex). May play a role in resolving emotional conflict as determined by functional magnetic resonance imaging.

CRP (C-reactive protein). A protein found in the blood plasma, whose levels increase during periods of inflammation in the body.

cuneus and precuneus. The cuneus is a smaller lobe in the occipital lobe that is involved in visual processing.

frontal limbic structures. Limbic areas in close proximity with the frontal lobes that support emotion, behavior, motivation, and long-term memory.

genome-wide association study. The examination of the entire genome to seek out genetic variants of SNPs (single-nucleotide polymorphisms) in different individuals.

inflammatory markers. In the presence of inflammation in the body, particular abnormal proteins may be released into the blood, and they can be identified by laboratory tests.

PTSD. Post-traumatic stress disorder.

SPECT scanning (single-photon emission computed tomography). A nuclear medicine imaging technique using gamma rays. It provides 3-D information.

temporal volumes (temporal lobes). Imaging and postmortem studies can be measured, and abnormalities, usually reductions, can be determined.

volumetric reductions. A range of prefrontal and subcortical volumetric abnormalities found in adolescents and adults with various psychiatric illnesses.

CHAPTER 23

Look at All the Mental Veterans

After serving in combat in the armed services, there is nothing veterans look forward to as much as being labeled *mental.* Whatever symptoms and sufferings they are enduring, being labeled mental by psychiatry is an automatic boost to their self-esteem, self-satisfaction, and well-being. Yes, that's what psychiatry tells them: *You* are mental, *you* are mental, and *you* are mental!

Two major illnesses veterans return with are TBI (traumatic brain injury) and PTSD (post-traumatic stress disorder). In TBI, the actual physical brain has been injured or damaged. In PTSD—a mental health problem, according to psychiatry—no comparable physical injury to the brain has occurred.

Those veterans are obviously in an emotional pit of self-indulgence. They would benefit from reintroduction to basic training, in which they would have real problems to consider.

Are you saying there are actual structural brain changes in PTSD? Then maybe the soldiers with PTSD will not need to be reintroduced into basic training to get over it and get on with it. Perhaps they aren't in an emotional pit of self-indulgence. Perhaps they have real symptoms based on actual brain abnormalities. Perhaps PTSD is not a mental health problem! But who dares say that to therapy psychiatrists? One can be very nervous challenging their authority by saying PTSD is not a mental health problem! After all, they are the experts in all the symptoms and illnesses under their jurisdiction, which are all mental health problems (according to *The Diagnostic and Statistical Manual of Mental Disorders*). Have you ever met an infuriated therapy psychiatrist?

PTSD is associated with marked reductions in gray matter in several brain areas. The extent of overall gray matter loss is equivalent to that found in severe, recurrent MDD. There is much overlap in the brain areas affected in both disorders and some differences. Gray matter is an essential brain ingredient that contains neurons and supporting cells that account for our higher brain functions and emotional well-being. Loss of gray matter equals loss of neurons!

In PTSD, the symptom of anxiety is inversely associated with reduced temporal volumes. In MDD, anxiety symptoms are associated with reduced volumes in the cuneus and precuneus. In addition to these findings (worked out with structural magnetic imaging scans), both disorders share volume reductions in frontal-limbic structures and the ACC (rostral anterior cingulate cortex). In PTSD, relative to MDD, there may be less volumetric reductions in the hippocampus.

The critical point is PTSD is associated with structural brain abnormalities[120] and not just TBI (traumatic brain injury). PTSD does not just arise in the context of mental turmoil evoked by stirring up those deeply buried conflicts in the id and superego by traumatic events. It is associated with genetic abnormalities.

How can a mental health problem have any association with genes? So far, therapy psychiatry has not yet claimed genes associated with mental illness are mental as opposed to physical genes.

In a genome-wide association study, the complete genomes of a large number of individuals are scanned, looking to identify genetic variations associated with different diseases. The largest such study

---

[120] Marjin C, et. al. "Structural brain abnormalities common to post-traumatic stress disorder and depression," *Journal of Psychiatry and Neuroscience.* July 2011, 364, 256–265.

of PTSD was completed in 2016.[121] It involved a very large sample of veterans, 3,167 with PTSD, and as a control group, 4,607 individuals who also had experienced major trauma but did not develop PTSD. The study, entitled the "New Soldier Study" (NSS) ran during 2011–2012. The objective was to identify SNPs associated with PTSD. There follows an explanation of them. What are single nucleotide polymorphisms (SNPs)?

Single nucleotide polymorphisms, frequently called SNPs (pronounced snips), are the most common type of genetic variation among people. Each SNP represents a difference in a single DNA building block, called a nucleotide. For example, a SNP may replace the nucleotide cytosine (C) with the nucleotide thymine (T) in a certain stretch of DNA.

SNPs occur normally throughout a person's DNA. They occur once in every three hundred nucleotides on average, which means there are roughly ten million SNPs in the human genome. Most commonly, these variations are found in the DNA between genes. They can act as biological markers, helping scientists locate genes that are associated with disease. When SNPs occur within a gene or in a regulatory region near a gene, they may play a more direct role in disease by affecting the gene's function.

Most SNPs have no effect on health or development. Some of these genetic differences, however, have proven to be very important in the study of human health. Researchers have found SNPs that may help predict an individual's response to certain drugs, susceptibility to environmental factors such as toxins, and risks of developing particular diseases. SNPs can also be used to track the inheritance of disease genes within families. Future studies will work to identify

[121] "Genome-wide Association Studies of Posttraumatic Stress Disorder in 2 Cohorts of U.S. Army Soldiers." Stein, Murray B., et al. *JAMA Psychiatry.* 2016; 73 7 695–704.

SNPs associated with complex diseases such as heart disease, diabetes, and cancer.[122]

The soldiers were studied in two major groupings according to race: African-Americans and individuals of European descent. In the former group, a significant locus (SNP) for PTSD was found on the ANKRD 55 gene on chromosome 5. In the second group, a significant locus (SNP) was found near the ZNF626 gene on chromosome 19. These genetic loci are closely associated with genes that are operative in a number of diseases. The genes for rheumatoid arthritis and psoriasis (both immunological diseases) are very closely related.

Therapy psychiatrists violently refute this. How could grubby physical symptoms like severe rashes or swollen painful joints have the remotest association with mental illness, in which complex, hard-to-understand, deep conflicts in the id and superego require psychoanalytic psychotherapy conducted brilliantly to understand their origins and produce a cure?

There is substantial evidence of immune system dysfunction in PTSD. Inflammatory markers are elevated, including CRP (C-reactive protein). Also, PTSD is associated with an increased incidence of real, physical symptoms and illnesses: cardiovascular disease, inflammatory bowel disease, and multiple sclerosis, for example.

For our soldiers, particularly those who have been in combat, what kind of treatment are they receiving in the mental health care system? A study published in ***Psychiatric Services*** investigated this.[123] Two studies were reviewed. The first screened for PTSD in 45,462 soldiers returning from Afghanistan from January 1 through December 31, 2010, who had been deployed in active-duty combat operations. Afghanistan veterans were chosen over Iraq veterans because there was relatively more combat there. Of this cohort, all who received

---

[122] *Genetics Home Reference: Your Guide to Understanding Genetic Conditions.* NIH. US National Library of Medicine.

[123] "PTSD treatment for soldiers after combat deployment: low utilization of mental health care and reasons for dropout. Hoge C. W., et al. *Psychiatric Services* Aug. 1, 2014; 65(8): 997–1004.

mandatory Post-Deployment Health Assessments (PDHA), 2,230 soldiers were diagnosed with PTSD within ninety days of leaving the combat zones. In the second study of an infantry brigade, also deployed in active combat zones, out of 2,876 soldiers, 229 were diagnosed with PTSD. The authors evaluated the adequacy of treatment for soldiers suffering from PTSD.[124]

The four main PTSD symptom clusters of the DSM-5 criteria are listed below:

- Intrusion. Examples include nightmares, unwanted thoughts of the traumatic events, flashbacks, and reacting to traumatic reminders with emotional distress or excessive physiological reactivity.
- Avoidance. Examples include avoiding triggers for traumatic memories including places, conversations, or other reminders.
- Negative alterations in cognitions and mood. Examples include distorted blame of self or others for the traumatic event, negative beliefs about oneself or the world, persistent negative emotions (e.g., fear, guilt, shame), feeling alienated, and constricted affect (e.g., inability to experience positive emotions).
- Alterations in arousal and reactivity. Examples include angry, reckless, or self-destructive behavior, sleep problems, concentration problems, increased startle response, and hypervigilance.

They were evaluating the level of utilization of available treatment for PTSD, the adequacy of treatment, and the reasons soldiers dropped out before completing treatment. Three previous studies were suggestive of underutilization of services, only a third receiving treatment for PTSD. These studies suggested soldiers are inhibited from seeking treatment because of negative attitudes toward mental

[124] "PTSD: National Guide to Medications for PTSD," Jeffreys, Matt, MD.

health care, the stigma associated with identifying as mentally ill, and a general disbelief in the efficacy of mental health treatment.)

The researchers defined minimally adequate treatment as at least eight sessions with a provider in a year. Of the 2,230 soldiers diagnosed with PTSD from the large cohort, only 41 percent received barely adequate care as defined by the eight-session metric. Of the 229 soldiers diagnosed with PTSD from the infantry brigade of 2,876 soldiers, only 17 percent received minimally adequate care; the balance received no care or an insufficient number of sessions. (If treatment for PTSD is adequate, for soldiers who complete a course of it, 70–80 percent show substantial improvement.) Overall, however, due to avoidance of treatment and high dropout rates, less than 33 percent have significant symptomatic and functional improvement. The soldiers' responses indicated a number of reasons for not seeking needed treatment or dropping out before completion. Among these were scheduling difficulties, a belief care would be or was ineffective, stigma associated with mental health treatment, and perceptions the professional was not suitably caring, communicative, or competent.[125] The authors summarize:

> This study represents a call to action to develop and test interventions to improve perceptions of mental health care and treatment engagement and retention in military, VHA, and civilian treatment settings. Dropping out of care is clearly the most important predictor of treatment failure; therefore, the most promising strategies to improve efficacy of evidence-based treatments will be those that address engagement, therapeutic rapport, and retention. Particular attention is needed to better understand the modifiable organizational, patient, and clinician factors and specific actions that clinicians and health care systems can take. Interventions related

---

[125] Ibid.

> to organizational barriers include ensuring adequate appointment availability and duration at convenient times and locations, as well as peer-to-peer outreach. Strategies to address patients' beliefs about treatment should consider perceptions of self-reliance (for example through motivational interviewing techniques). Policies concerning confidentiality, especially for treatment of comorbid substance use disorders, remain an ongoing issue in the military. Clinician factors that warrant close examination concern the skills and training needed to optimally foster patient-centered care.

The Department of Veterans Affairs tabulated 7403 veterans died by suicide in 2014.[126] (This statistic may understate the total, as many veterans are not treated by the V.A. The suicide rate was highest for young soldiers between eighteen and twenty-nine. The rate for veterans is seven times higher than for the general population. Two major disorders account for many of these deaths: PTSD and TBI.

In more than 50 percent of soldiers, the two disorders are comorbid and often compounded by MDD. This heavy symptomatic load is often accompanied by despair, a sense of futility, and an inability to lead a normal life. As already touched on, these veterans are often reluctant to seek help, in particular viewing PTSD and depression as not real brain illnesses, but indicative of failure of character, warranting a sense of shame and guilt. This reluctance is reinforced by a disbelief therapies can be helpful and fear of medications.

Of course, PTSD is a brain disorder deserving of the best treatment, but since the symptoms of PTSD are usually comingled with the symptoms of TBI, the latter also remains poorly evaluated and treated. PTSD and TBI have a large overlap of symptoms: insomnia, pain, headaches, irritability, poor concentration, memory difficulties,

---

[126] "Twenty veterans a day committed suicide in 2014, new data show." Zoroya, Gregg. *USA Today*, July 7, 2016.

anhedonia, and social isolation. For those who ultimately seek treatment, the commonality of symptoms often leads to diagnostic confusion on the part of the often poorly trained mental health practitioner, resulting in missed diagnosis and perpetuation of the disability. There is a possible bright spot in improving accuracy of diagnosis of both and discriminating between the two disorders and/or if comorbid.

Theodore A. Henderson, MD, PhD, reporting in the September 2015 issue of *Brain Imaging and Behavior*, has been able to greatly increase the accuracy of diagnosis using SPECT scanning, claiming scans identify definite differences between PTSD and TBI, making it possible to distinguish them one from the other and both from comorbid TBI.

SPECT is a purely physical (radiological) diagnostic resource. How many therapists and therapy psychiatrists will be aware of it, know how to refer for it, or know what to do with the data the scans elicit?

GLOSSARY

adrenocorticoids. Any of the hormones produced by the adrenal cortex, including cortisol, aldosterone, and androgens.

amygdalae. A set of neurons linked to fear and pleasure responses.

cAMP. Protein kinase family members regulate numerous cellular responses such as gene expression, cell proliferation, and inflammation. Activation of these enzymes requires phosphorylation facilitated by cAMP.

amine neurotransmitters. An important grouping of neurotransmitters having a more complex protein structure and upon which drugs act (serotonin, dopamine, and others).

anticonvulsants. Reduce the excitability of nervous tissue. Used in treatment of epilepsy and bipolar disorder.

apoptosis. A built-in program of neurons, which if triggered by certain conditions, causes the neuron to destroy itself.

atypical antipsychotic. A newer generation of antipsychotics, generally having reduced side effects with a wide variety of uses beyond psychosis.

BDNF. A neurotrophic factor sustaining neuron health.

benzodiazepines. A class of psychoactive drugs that enhances the activity of the neurotransmitter, GABA, at a specific site at its receptor. It has antianxiety actions.

double-blind randomized controlled studies. A type of scientific experiment or study designed to reduce bias when developing a new treatment.

executive functioning. Promotes adaptive adjustment to one's environment, responsibilities, and relationships.

FOS-JUN combination protein. A critical protein for the cell cycle due to its regulation of transcription of genes.

GABA-A receptor. It binds gamma-amino-butyric acid. The major inhibitory neurotransmitter in the nervous system.

GABA-B receptor agonist. A drug that stimulates a subtype of GABA receptor by binding to it.

genes, early/late. Early genes, when activated by the relevant transcription factors, activate the late genes, which are the workhorses of cell building and maintenance.

glucocorticoid receptor. Binds cortisol and other glucocorticoids.

glutamate. An amino acid neurotransmitter with a generally excitatory effect on neurons.

G-protein-linked cascade. One of four systems transmitting signals from receptors on the cell membrane to inside the cell to reach the genes in the cell nucleus.

hypothalamic-pituitary-adrenal axis. A complex of three endocrine glands producing steroid hormones involved in the stress reaction.

ion channel. Pores formed of proteins in cell membrane that control passage of ions into and out of neurons.

lithium. Lithium salts are used in the treatment of mood disorders.

MAOI antidepressant. A type of antidepressant that may have efficacy if more commonly used drugs fail. Requires experienced prescriber to prevent serious side effects.

Mini Neuropsychiatric Interview. A printed series of scales requiring patient response. Takes fifteen minutes to complete. Greatly clarifies psychiatric diagnosis and differential diagnosis.

mood stabilizer. Also known as anticonvulsants and used to treat epilepsy and bipolar disorders.

neuromodulator. A physiological process in which a given neuron uses one or more chemicals to regulate diverse populations of neurons.

neuropeptide. Small protein molecules that can act like neurotransmitters.

neurotrophic factor. A family of biomolecules that are peptides or small proteins that support neuron health.

prefrontal cortical functions. This brain region is the location of higher cognitive functions, planning, decision-making, moderating social behavior, and adoptive judgements.

pre/post synaptic neuron/receptor. In each case, involving the first neuron initiating a mechanism or action in a second neuron.

presynaptic alpha-2 adrenergic inhibitory auto receptor for norepinephrine. It inhibits noradrenaline and 5-hydroxytryptamine release in the cerebral cortex as learned in experiments with rats.

QT-prolongation. Abnormality on EKG that can lead to possibly fatal cardiac arrhythmia. Prescriber experience is essential.

serotonin reuptake inhibitor (SSRI) antidepressant. They block the presynaptic serotonergic neuron from taking unused serotonin back inside the cell to be used again.

serotonin-noradrenergic reuptake inhibitor (SNRI). In addition to blocking serotonin reuptake, also blocks the reuptake of noradrenaline back into noradrenergic neurons.

serotonin transport. The movement of serotonin molecules both within neurons, in between neurons in the synapse, and also back into neurons.

signal-transduction cascade. Signal relay pathways from one neuron through a synapse to a second neuron, ultimately permitting communication between their respective genomes (genes).

synapse. The delicate structure through which neurons communicate with one another by means of neurotransmitters.

TBI. Traumatic brain injury.

tricyclic antidepressant. The oldest type of antidepressant. It remains in use for certain patients. Prescriber should be experienced with them to monitor for potential serious side effects.

ventricular arrhythmia. A potentially fatal arrhythmia of the heart that can be fatal. Tricyclic antidepressants can be implicated if the prescriber is inexperienced in their prescription and unfamiliar with their side effects or effect on the EKG.

CHAPTER 24

Expertise and PTSD/TBI

Evidence-Based Practice (From Wikipedia)

> Evidence-based practice (EBP) is an interdisciplinary approach to clinical practice that has been gaining ground following its formal introduction in 1992. It started in medicine as evidence-based medicine (EBM) and spread to other fields such as audiology, speech-language pathology, dentistry, nursing, psychology, social work, education, library and information science. EBP is traditionally defined in terms of a three-legged stool integrating three basic principles: (1) the best available research evidence bearing on whether and why a treatment works (2) clinical expertise (clinical judgment and experience) to rapidly identify each patient's unique health state and diagnosis, their individual risks and benefits of potential treatments, and (3) client preferences and values.

Evidence-based practice must strive to go far beyond the bare-bones diagnostic and treatment services of minimally adequate treatment (which of course is better than no treatment or totally inadequate treatment). What should the characteristics of comprehensive treatment be, and what practitioners can actually provide it? (You would think veterans would deserve no less).

The two clinical avenues for treatment of PTSD are pharmacological and psychotherapeutic. Can't any therapy psychiatrist write a prescription for 10 mg of Prozac? Can't any therapist just sit down with a veteran and by bantering and talking back and forth, relieve the veteran's symptoms. Everyone knows about Prozac. Everyone knows about the therapy shrink (MSW, PhD, therapy psychiatrist).

Well, maybe just prescribing a little Prozac isn't enough. Maybe light psychotherapeutic discussion is inadequate. However, that's what the bulk of veterans receive—the ones who get any treatment at all). That is the hallmark of the current mental health care system.

Psychopharmacology[127]

The average therapy psychiatrist who happens to diagnose PTSD will prescribe one dose of whatever antidepressant he or she is used to—maybe Prozac 20 mg—and most likely leave it at that, while also insisting the patient come for a weekly psychotherapy session for an indeterminate amount of time. The therapy is generally a form of loosely administered nonspecific form of psychoanalytic psychotherapy for which there is little evidence for efficacy in PTSD.

Generally, the therapy psychiatrist does not use measurement scales to quantify symptoms, evaluate for comorbidities (ADHD, panic disorder, etc.), or measure how symptoms respond to treatment procedures. In contrast, a good internist will always take measurements before starting treatment, for example, of hypertension. These will include baseline measurements of blood pressure and then ongoing measurements to see how treatment is impacting on blood pressure. Ultimately, the objective is to bring the blood pressure to normal levels. The internist will always be on the lookout for other illnesses the patient may have in addition to hypertension by ordering and

---

[127] "PTSD: National Center for PTSD." Jeffries, Matt, Clinicians Guide to Medications for PTSD.

following up with relevant laboratory examinations (*differential diagnosis*). The internist also will never prescribe a low dose of a blood pressure medication and just leave it at that. He will draw from a number of classes of blood pressure medications raised to a treatment dose level requiring titration and monitoring along the way, and in difficult cases, may use combinations of classes of blood pressure medications—even up to three different classes—to reach the therapeutic objective of normalized blood pressure.

Well, the pharmacological treatment of all the major psychiatric disorders should follow an identical path—a path the average therapy psychiatrist is unable to replicate due to ignorance about neuroscience and the complex, sophisticated psychopharmacology that must be based on an understanding of neuroscience. Does the therapy psychiatrist know what a synapse is or what the functions of a synapse are? That so-called mental illnesses may adversely affect synapse integrity and functioning? The approximate number of synapses in the brain? What apoptosis is? What a neurotrophic factor is? What BDNF is? What recognition molecules are? What a dendrite is? The approximate number of neurotransmitter types in the brain? What are the chief amine neurotransmitters? The differences between pre and postsynaptic neurons? What a signal-transduction cascade is? What first, second, third, and fourth messengers do? What the four major types of signal-transduction cascades are? The key messenger molecules for the G-protein-linked cascade? What an ion channel is? What the functions of ion channels are? What early genes do? What late genes do? What the Fos-Jun combination protein is—and its functions?

This series of questions could continue for pages. Is the psychiatrist a neurobiologically informed clinician? For the average therapy psychiatrist, the categorical answer is no! (More on this later).

Well, what does expert pharmacological treatment consist of? First, measurement of symptoms and differential diagnosis. One excellent series of measurement scales to accomplish this is the utilization of the Mini-Neuropsychiatric Interview or alternative measurement-scales at the time of the initial evaluation. Then periodic measurements taken during the course of treatment. How many therapy psychiatrists utilize scales? Virtually none. An apt metaphor would be an internist treating hypertension but never taking a blood pressure measurement because he thinks the patient looks like he has hypertension, then prescribing his one dose of one blood pressure medication, and then in follow-up concluding the patient looks like his blood pressure is improved, again without actually taking a blood pressure measurement!

In order to treat soldiers with PTSD, a wide variety of mediations from different classes may be necessary. It is critical to titrate each medication carefully to avoid adverse side effects, to raise them to effective dosage levels, and if combining medications, to be aware of potential drug interactions and side effects. In other words, pill prescribing is inadequate. Advanced pharmacological skills and experience is mandatory. Matt Jeffreys, MD[128] explains this complex process, and the following comments are extracted from his article:

> The competent clinician must realize each case of PTSD has unique biological, psychological, and social determinants, so treatment must be individualized. The clinician should be aware of what scientific evidence supports a given clinical decision to prescribe.

This means awareness of double-blind, randomized, controlled studies that support the clinical decision. He must also be aware that referral to evidence-based psychotherapy may add synergistic benefit to pharmacological treatment, such as CBT, prolonged exposure (PE) therapy, or cognitive processing therapy (CPT). The competent clinician should at least make an effort to locate such qualified therapists in his community.

---

128 "Clinicians Guide to Medications for PTSD," PTSD: National Center for PTSD.

The current evidence base for PTSD pharmacology supports the SSRIs and venlafaxine (Effexor), both a serotonergic and noradrenergic reuptake inhibitor. In some cases, additional medication types may be necessary and prescribed off label. The prescriber must conduct a differential diagnosis to rule out other disorders that might be adversely affected by the prescription of an antidepressant alone. An example would be forms of bipolar disorder, in which an antidepressant could trigger a severe manic episode, causing gross disruption of the patient's life, trigger an outbreak of illegal behavior, or necessitate emergency hospitalization. In such patients, the antidepressant should only be prescribed after the patient is on an effective dose of lithium or an anticonvulsant (mood stabilizer). The prescription of such medications requires clinical expertise and medical knowledge.

The prescriber should be a brain psychiatrist and be aware of the medication's effect on the brain, the fear-anxiety-mood circuitry, and upon the levels of particularly the neuroamine neurotransmitters, serotonin, norepinephrine, dopamine, glutamate, gamma-amino butyric acid, and acetylcholinergic.

As for measurement, the MINI-Neuropsychiatric Interview covers all the bases. Another scale, the Clinician-Administered PTSD Scale, is the gold standard for initial PTSD evaluation. A shorter scale, the Post-Traumatic Stress Disorder Checklist (PCL-5) is useful for follow-up measurement of symptoms.

The prescriber should have knowledge, in so far as it is available, of how medications impact on the underlying neurobiology of PTSD. An example is knowing that some patients have a deficiency in amygdalae serotonin transport and that SSRIs can modulate both peripheral and central nervous system, serotonergic neurotransmission.

It may be necessary to change this basic serotonergic treatment approach depending on side effects, response, comorbidities, and patient preferences. Additional examples, in addition to the presence of bipolar disorder, would be intolerable sexual side effects or gastrointestinal side effects due to elevated serotonin levels. The maximum benefit from SSRI treatment will be dependent on achieving adequate dosage and an adequate duration of treatment and keeping a close eye on whether the patient is adhering to treatment.

For each of the SSRIs (sertraline, paroxetine, fluoxetine) among others, it is critical to know their dosage ranges and side effect profiles. If a prescribed SSRI, after adequate titration and duration of treatment, fails to yield significant symptomatic relief, then prescription of other types of antidepressants may be necessary. The prescriber must be skilled at tapering the SSRI and cautiously starting and titrating the second antidepressant upward. One such alternative antidepressant is mirtazapine, which has a unique mechanism of action affecting both serotonin and norepinephrine through blockade of the presynaptic alpha-2 adrenergic inhibitory autoreceptor for norepinephrine and the blockade of postsynaptic 5-HT2 and 5-HT3 serotonergic receptors. Bupropion (Wellbutrin-brand) is one of the most commonly prescribed antidepressants because it does not cause sexual side effects or drowsiness. Unfortunately, it does not work for PTSD!

On occasion, a severely symptomatic veteran (or civilian) with PTSD will fail to respond to the antidepressants, making it essential the psychiatrist is familiar and experienced in the prescription of anticonvulsants, just as the average neurologist is. They affect the balance between glutamate, an excitatory neurotransmitter, and GABA (gamma-aminobutyric acid), an inhibitory one. There are several different anticonvulsants, carbamazepine (Tegretol), divalproex (Depakote), lamotrigine (Lamictal), and topiramate (Topamax), among others. All of these are also prescribed for psychiatric disorders. A recent meta-analysis showed strong support for the use of topiramate for PTSD, demonstrating efficacy comparable to paroxetine (Paxil, an SSRI), but of course having an entirely different mechanism of action from SSRIs.

- Carbamazepine (Tegretol). Requires monitoring of white blood cell counts due to risk of agranulocytosis. Will self-induce its own metabolism and increase the metabolism of other medications, including oral contraceptives.

- Divalproex (Depakote). Requires monitoring of liver function tests due to risk of hepatotoxicity and platelet levels due to risk of thrombocytopenia. Target dosage is ten times the patient's weight in pounds.
- Lamotrigine (Lamictal). Requires slow titration according to the package insert due to risk of serious rash.
- Topiramate (Topamax). Requires clinical monitoring for glaucoma, sedation, dizziness, and ataxia.

In order to prescribe these drugs safely, the prescriber must be a real physician.

In particular cases, the prescription of an atypical antipsychotic may be necessary. This class of drugs, originally developed for psychotic disorders, is now prescribed in a wide variety of illnesses, including neurological and medical ones. In the case of PTSD, the prescriber must be able to detect (careful examination, history taking, and differential diagnosis) psychotic symptomatology, which may be subtle and for which an atypical antipsychotic may be critical if overall improvement is to occur. Again, appropriate selection of an atypical and then careful titration with awareness of potential side effects and drug interactions are necessary. The prescriber must be aware atypicals should not be prescribed alone for PTSD, but in selected cases along with other medications.

Additional classes of medication may be of use. Tricyclic antidepressants or an MAOI inhibitor-type antidepressant may benefit some veterans. Tricyclics can cause cardiac arrhythmias through QT prolongation, especially in overdose, which can result in fatal ventricular arrhythmias. MAOIs can result in fatal episodes of stroke or serotonin syndrome (when levels of serotonin build up too high in the brain). If one of such medications can control a veteran's symptoms—permitting a return to a normal symptom-reduced life—the prescription may be justified. (They can be used safely if the prescriber is a brain psychiatrist, well-trained in, and experienced in their prescription).

Another medication, prazosin, is actually a blood pressure medication, a postsynaptic alpha-adrenergic blocker. There is substantial evidence, apart from lowering blood pressure, that it also reduces the intensity of nightmares and terrors in PTSD, promoting restorative sleep. It also may reduce alcohol cravings in veterans with PTSD who have comorbid alcohol use disorder, supporting abstinence or reduced consumption.

Other medications that may be useful for PTSD are buspirone and beta-blockers used adjunctively for the treatment of hyperarousal symptoms. Buspirone is an agonist at the presynaptic serotonin 5-HT1A receptor and a partial agonist at the postsynaptic 5-HT1A receptor. Beta-blockers, which are used to treat cardiovascular disorders, particularly hypertension, block norepinephrine at synapses in the central nervous system and adrenaline within organs of the body, muscles, sweat glands, and the heart.

Benzodiazepines enhance the therapeutic (and side) effects at the GABA-A receptor in the central nervous system. It is generally felt, in most cases, to avoid anything but very short-term use, up to five days, of this class in PTSD, but then the experienced clinician should not make absolute categorical rules. Some veterans with comorbid PTSD and severe panic disorder may greatly benefit from careful long-term prescription of benzodiazepines. Examples of this class are lorazepam (Ativan), clonazepam (Klonopin), alprazolam (Xanax), and diazepam (Valium). The key to successful prescription of these again is a broad-based knowledge of and experience in pharmacology. Generally, the first three are preferable to Valium.

So, it should be obvious that PTSD is a complex brain disorder—not a mental health problem—with many specific biological mechanisms that can be beneficially targeted by a wide variety of medications. However, it is even more complicated. There are additional dysregulated brain mechanisms that may be pharmacologically targeted in the future by new classes of medications.

The multifaceted, complex neurobiological dysregulations in PTSD may open the way to additional varied pharmacological approaches.

These neurobiological disturbances can be conceptualized in part as a dysregulation of the hypothalamic-pituitary-adrenal (HPA) axis and an imbalance between excitatory and inhibitory brain neurocircuitry, especially of adrenergic mechanisms. Patients with PTSD have abnormal HPA function—compared to patients without PTSD—and much greater variations in their levels of adrenocorticoids. Therefore, the brain's fear circuitry exhibits excessive activation overriding prefrontal cortical functions such as executive planning and the capacity to keep perspective through making rational judgments.

Even minor stresses trigger the brain's adrenergic circuitry and the associated frontal cortical dysfunctions, as well as peripheral symptoms in the body such as sweating, tremors, rapid heart rate, and sensations associated with emotional terror. The impact on the prefrontal cortex can be described as a *freeze response.*

One new approach for treatment rests on the hypothesis of *glucocorticoid dysregulation* during and after trauma via its influence on the HPA axis, which might be a treatment target. The glucocorticoid receptors in the brain modulate the effects of stress, and perhaps through this route, the symptoms of PTSD might be ameliorated. Early interventions with cortisol give preliminary evidence that it reduces symptoms. In one study, cortisol administered prior to prolonged exposure therapy demonstrated significantly better retention of treatment. Several actions of glucocorticoids include potentiating glutamate at NMDA receptors, decreased intensity of fear memories, and beneficial interactions with the noradrenergic circuitry.

Two neuropeptides appear to play a role in PTSD, substance P and neuropeptide-Y (NPY). Some combat troops exposed to the stress of combat have lowered levels of NPY, but resilient Special Forces troops exhibit elevated levels! A potential therapeutic avenue might be to potentiate NPY, which is a neuromodulator.

A related substance is the neuropeptide oxytocin. Preliminary trials have demonstrated intranasal administration of oxytocin results in a decrease in arousal symptoms. D-cycloserine (DCS) is a partial agonist of the glutamatergic N-methyl-D-aspartate (NMDA) receptor.

Based on animal research, it is hypothesized use of DCS as an adjunct to exposure (psycho) therapy may reduce the number of sessions required. Another study suggests methylphenidate, a stimulant medication used to treat ADHD, improved cognitive complaints, as well as PTSD symptom severity in both TBI and PTSD. Larger studies are needed.

Ketamine, the anesthetic agent, modulates the balance between glutamate and GABA at the NMDA receptor and serotonergic activity at 5HT receptors. A recent trial showed benefits in PTSD, although problematic issues are limited duration of action beyond two or three weeks and the potential for abuse. Newer ketamine analogs could lead to treatment options independent from serotonin and norepinephrine-based treatment.

The endocannabinoid systems are another potential treatment avenue. Abnormalities at cannabinoid receptors coupled with reduced levels of anandamide (an endogenous cannabinoid) have been found in PTSD patients. Marijuana, a direct agonist of the cannabinoid type 1 receptor, is obviously not a viable therapeutic option, but indirect influencing of this pathway may have therapeutic potential. Baclofen is used clinically as a muscle relaxant and is a GABA-B receptor agonist. A small study employing it in conjunction with an SSRI, citalopram, demonstrated significant reduction of symptoms in comparison to citalopram and a placebo.

It should be obvious at this point that PTSD is a brain-based illness caused by a multiplicity of physical deregulations. Why do the therapy psychiatrists still adamantly insist it is a mental health problem? Could it be they have brain freeze of their collective prefrontal cortices?

The article outlines common barriers to successful pharmacological treatment of PTSD, of which several areas are mentioned. There should be sufficient time in a pharmacological appointment to discuss potential side effects, weigh the risks and benefits of the selected medication or medications, and describe the likely dosage levels to achieve benefits and the likely duration of treatment. The importance of close adherence to the prescription must be explained, and some of the more routine negative attitudes anticipated include fear of side effects, including sexual side effects, viewing medications as a crutch or a sign of weak character, an exaggerated fear of becoming addicted to medication, not understanding the medication must be taken on a regular schedule, confusing medications, and missing doses. Of course, it is the clinician's responsibility to assess if the patient is self-medicating with alcohol or street drugs. Prescribing physicians need to understand patients with PTSD may have an extra sensitivity to side effects, so it is important to cautiously start and increase dosage and to be aware of potential interactions with other medications the patient may be taking.

Pharmacotherapy for serious PTSD is not for amateurs. Such clinicians need broad experience with prescribing for PTSD.

Psychotherapy

Especially important is a PTSD-specific psychological assessment and therapeutic approach. Peter Gutierrez, a clinical research psychologist at Denver VA Medical Center,[129] states veterans who sustained a TBI or developed PTSD or both in combination, are particularly vulnerable to suicidality. Identifying those at risk is of primary importance.

Veterans are much more likely to use firearms for suicidal purposes. He does not ask whether they have a weapon, but how many they own and where they are kept to assess the ease of access. It is critical to clarify you are not going to confiscate the weapons and to reassure them. "I am not talking about taking your gun away. I am helping you keep safe in a time of crisis."

He describes one veteran who slept with a gun under his pillow because it was the only way he felt safe. If there is apparent serious risk of a suicide attempt, he will involve family members or friends who agree to take temporary charge of the weapons. If absolutely necessary, he will consider hospitalization, but he will first attempt

---

[129] Yasgur, M, MA, LSW, "Suicide, Prevention in Veterans," *Psychiatry Advisor*, June 22, 2016.

more frequent appointments, telephone contacts, and a safety plan involving relatives and friends if feasible.

In order to conduct beneficial therapeutic discussion with a veteran, it is important to become aware of the details of his service, in what theaters he served, what injuries he sustained, and what particular combat experiences he encountered. Both TBI and PTSD affect executive functioning, and veterans usually present with impairments in problem-solving skills and stress tolerance, a depletion of cognitive resources resulting in decreases in working memory, and reduced abilities to navigate a variety of demands and stresses in the environment: pain, medical procedures, employment or lack thereof, and interpersonal conflicts. Then, treatment must be tailored according to the veteran's individual needs based on his ability to process information, make decisions, and engage in planning.[130]

The current mental health care system is a totally inadequate venue to competently diagnose and treat veterans with PTSD. What is required is a treatment system that will deliver the sophisticated, specialized pharmacological and psychotherapeutic services that have just been described—and to do so on a predictable basis!

[130] Dr. Gutierrez also frequently refers his veterans (he is a doctor of psychology) for additional neurological and neuropsychiatric evaluation.

GLOSSARY

allosteric modulation. A substance that indirectly influences (or modulates) the effects of an agonist or inverse agonist at a receptor.

antibodies. A large protein used by the immune system to identify and destroy pathogens like bacteria and viruses.

anti-inflammatory agents. Some common ones like aspirin and NAC (n-acetylcysteine) may prevent brain damage in schizophrenia if used at an early state of the disease.

aspirin. If used in the earliest stages of schizophrenia—generally ten years before the outbreak of psychotic symptoms—it could prevent serious symptoms and brain damage.

catabolism. The process of breaking down larger molecules, usually to release energy from foods.

cognitive symptoms. Present in the early stages of schizophrenia. Disturbances of thinking processes characterized by negative or disturbed thinking, difficulty concentrating, forgetfulness, distractibility, memory loss, and indecisiveness.

cytokines. A category of small proteins that are important in cell signaling and inflammatory processes.

dopaminergic neurotransmission abnormalities. According to imaging studies, there is increased dopamine turnover in schizophrenia.

dorsolateral prefrontal cortex. An area of the prefrontal cortex with numerous connections to other brain areas. It is known for its involvement in higher cognitive functions, including working memory, cognitive flexibility, and planning.

early-stage disease in schizophrenia. This starts ten years before the outbreak of obvious psychotic symptoms when the disease is much more treatable. Unfortunately, it is almost never diagnosed at that point in the current mental health care system.

estrogens. If employed in women with early stage schizophrenia, may prevent the full-blown illness. However, this almost never occurs in the current mental health care system.

free radicals. Any atom or molecule that has a single unpaired electron in its outer shell. Free radicals are highly reactive and can cause oxidative damage to biological structures in the brain. They may promote more rapid aging of tissue. Caloric restriction and healthy DNA repair may counteract.

GABA (gamma-amino-butyric acid). An important inhibitory neurotransmitter, particularly of glutamate.

GABA a5. A subunit of the GABA receptor.

GABA-ergic medications. GABA agonists promote activity of the receptor and can be associated with antianxiety and anticonvulsant actions. If the dosage prescribed is too high, they can cause sedation as a side effect.

GABA-ergic neurotransmission. A major neurotransmitter system for GABA.

GABA interneuron. Inhibitory neurons playing a vital role in neural circuitry and activity. Reduced activity in schizophrenia results in less inhibitory modulation of glutamate and dopamine activity, which can worsen symptoms.

GABA-A receptor. It binds the neurotransmitter gamma-amino-butyric acid as well as several exogenous drugs, including benzodiazepines, steroids, barbiturates, ethanol, and inhaled anesthetics.

genome-wide association studies. Also known as whole-genome association studies. It is an examination of a genome-wide set of genes for genetic variations in different individuals to see if any variant is associated with some particular trait. They focus on SNPs and diseases.

glial cells. Nonneuronal cells that provide support and protection for neurons and produce myelin, the protective coating for axons. They hold neurons in place, supply nutrients and oxygen, keep neurons separated, and destroy pathogens and dead neurons.

glutamatergic neurons. Neurons that synthesize and excrete glutamate.

glutamatergic neurotransmission. Glutamate is the most abundant neurotransmitter and the major excitatory one. In excess, it can become toxic to neural tissue (glutamate toxicity).

glutamatergic treatments. In mood disorders and schizophrenia, there are significant dysfunctions in glutamatergic mechanisms in which early treatment may prevent progression of the disease, but this rarely occurs in the current mental health care system.

glycine transporter. A membrane protein that recaptures glycine, a major inhibitory neurotransmitter. Also called a reuptake pump. One of its forms may support the NMDAr (receptor) and be a potential treatment for early-stage schizophrenia.

immunity markers in serum. Examples are C-reactive proteins and multiple additional molecules. If identified and measured, they can indicate the status of a given disease.

inflammatory processes of the brain. Low-grade inflammation is characteristic in schizophrenia and precedes the onset of the overt psychotic symptoms by ten years. By then, irreversible cognitive deficits and dysfunctions have occurred.

inverse agonist. An agonist is a neurotransmitter, which when it lands on its receptor, facilitates active, generally beneficial processes in the neuron. An inverse agonist reduces the effect of the agonist or silences it completely.

ketamine. An antagonist (shuts off activity) of the NMDA (receptor) that produces all the symptoms of schizophrenia.

kynurenic acid. A metabolic product of tryptophanic metabolism, which can have injurious properties in schizophrenia, perhaps by excessive activation of dopaminergic neurotransmission.

life charting. Use of a standardized forms and graphs to keep accurate track of the course of the symptoms of bipolar disorder over time.

mental health care system. Totally fails to recognize and properly treat early-stage disease when it is curable.

mesolimbic pathway. Participates in the reward system of the brain. A dopaminergic pathway associated with the mesolimbic brain areas.

MHC class I inflammatory molecules. Major histocompatibility-complex molecules. They interact with helper cells to produce a localized immune response against pathogens.

microglia. A type of immune cell in the brain.

microglia, activated. In this state, can produce neurotoxic substances that damage neurons, axons, and glial cells, resulting in cognitive symptoms.

n-acetylcysteine (NAC). If used in early-stage disease—approximately ten years before psychotic symptom onset—might prevent brain damage.

neurotoxic substances. Substances that damage neural tissue. Can have endogenous sources (activated microglial cells) or exogenous sources (ketamine toxins).

N-methyl-D-aspartate receptor (NMDAr). Felt to have weakened efficacy in schizophrenia.

NMDAr agonists. Molecules, which upon binding to the NMDAr, will improve its level of activity.

phencyclidine. An NMDAr antagonist that produces all the symptoms of schizophrenia—even in people without the disease.

polyunsaturated fatty acids. If utilized early in the disease process, could have many beneficial effects.

postmortem studies. The laboratory study of tissue taken from the brains of deceased individuals.

post-striatal dopamine receptors. A class of G-protein coupled receptors, D1 and DO. Implicated in motivation, cognition, pleasure, and memory and learning. They prevent loss of gray matter. The ultimate objective of successful treatment requires specialized intervention long before onset of psychotic symptoms.

psychotic symptoms. Very late-stage but obvious symptoms. When in the current mental health care system, the diagnosis is sometimes finally made, by then, irreversible brain damage has already occurred.

risk genes. Increase the risk of developing a disease. Single nucleotide polymorphisms (SNPs) can represent a slightly different structure, which can result in a nucleotide that can be a source of a harmful genetic variation, resulting in disease or harmful traits.

striatum. A subcortical part of the forebrain and a critical part of the rewards system. It receives glutamatergic and dopaminergic inputs from different sources and is the primary input into the basal ganglia system. It coordinates multiple aspects of cognition, including motor and action planning, decision-making, motivation, reinforcement, and reward perception.

superoxides. Molecules that are biologically toxic to invading organisms dependent on oxygen.

vagus nerve. The tenth cranial nerve with many branches and functions. It is a treatment target for Parkinson's disease and severe major depression.

CHAPTER 25

Final

Unfortunately, therapy psychiatry's resistance to becoming an authentic (real) medical specialty has reduced the authority of psychiatry. Its credibility is so lacking that other unusual parties claim to be experts in treating mental health problems. In this matter, therapy psychiatry directly permits the continued moth-eaten functioning of the so-called mental health care system and—through errors of commission—invites in squadrons of therapists with rather unusual ideas who set themselves up as experts in treating the mentally ill.

Unknowingly, hundreds of thousands of these mentally ill individuals are led down strange pathways, which retrogress back to the prescientific era. It has been mentioned previously that 70–80 percent of psychiatrists have little interest in brain mechanisms and their relationships to pharmacological actions. They went to medical school to pull down higher fees than social workers or psychologists, administering a rather banal, nonspecific, so-called psychodynamically oriented psychotherapy.

It's as if 80 percent of neurologists went to medical school to pull down higher fees than physical therapists for the practice of physical therapy rather than neurological medicine. NAMI,[131] the National Alliance on Mental Illness, which also needs a name change,

---

131 NAMI. The National Alliance on Mental Illness. 3803 N Fairfax Drive, Suite 100, Arlington, VA 22203.

has supplied statistics on the number of Americans impacted by so-called mental illness—about one in seventeen. About 13.6 million individuals have the most serious illnesses such as schizophrenia, major depression, and bipolar disorder.

Approximately 60 percent of affected adults and nearly half of youths ages eight to fifteen receive no mental health services. These illnesses strike young individuals; half having an onset by age four and three-quarters by age twenty-four. Despite the existence of effective treatments, selecting a really competent provider is just Russian roulette. It's hit or miss.

There are long delays, sometimes decades, between the first appearance of symptoms and when people get help. (Help? Welcome to Russian roulette.) Individuals with serious mental illness die on average of twenty-five years prematurely, which is largely due to treatable medical conditions.

You can be sure the average therapy psychiatrist is not vigilant enough to refer for medical evaluation and treatment. Since they basically reject the practice of medicine, they may ignore or gloss over real physical symptoms.

According to NAMI, more than 50 percent of students with a mental health conditions drop out of treatment, which is the highest dropout rate of any disability group. Suicide is the third-leading cause of death of young people between fifteen and twenty-four, and 90 percent have one or more mental disorders.

Veterans represent 20 percent of all suicides nationally. All these young people had their lives terminated before they even had a chance to learn who they are as they progressed through their lives. If Abraham Lincoln, who had two severe major depressive episodes in his early thirties, had suicided, who would have preserved the integrity of the United States during the Civil War?

Without a strong, unified America, where would the world be? It would be under the totalitarian control of Stalin, Hitler, and Tojo! Thank God his friends kept close watch over him, fastidiously removing all knives and other implements with which, if he had easy access, he could have killed himself in the midst of the deep freeze of a severe major depressive episode.

Care without Labels[132] (With Commentary by the Author in Parentheses)

Caroline began hearing voices in grade school. She remembers being very upset when at age thirteen, a psychiatrist told her if she didn't take her meds, her brain would become more and more damaged. This made her feel hopeless because the drugs just made her feel worse.

(Did the psychiatrist explain to her the scientific evidence of the benefits of medication? Did he start with too high a dose? Did he keep close contact by phone to inquire about side effects and reassure her?)

For the next ten years, she saw psychiatrists—and was hospitalized. She feels she was led down a rabbit hole of failed treatments.

(What in God's name were these psychiatrists doing?)

Most therapy psychiatrists do not like treating the most ill; they are uninteresting, they are incapable of deep psychoanalytic therapy to dig out the deepest conflicts in the id and superego, and so they a pill and spend as little time with them as possible. Since they have incomplete knowledge and little interest in real pharmacology, any pill will do. The patient's symptoms are a pain, so knock out the symptoms with large doses of poorly understood medications. Then add a few more. Ignore the patient's hints of side effects. If they're psychotic anyway, what's the difference if they have side effects?

Sarah had been hearing voices for years and became suicidal in college. She was given a diagnosis of borderline personality disorder and was placed on medications that had severe side effects. She was told by her psychiatrist that she was a ticking time bomb. "I'd never finish college … never have a job … never have kids, and always be on psychiatric medication."

***

[132] *New York Times*, Aug. 9, 2016.

Marty had been prescribed Thorazine.

(Thorazine is the absolutely most ancient, outmoded antipsychotic medication. Maybe his psychiatrist had learned to prescribe Thorazine in the 1950s and been ignoring the field of psychopharmacology and all the subsequent developments since then.)

Marty said all he could do was lay on the couch. He finally stopped Thorazine and refused all subsequent medications. These individuals and thousands of others are refugees from therapy-psychiatry. Instead they have joined an alternative kind of "mental" health care that is very much anti-mainstream, support groups for voice hearers, or HVN (Hearing Voices Network).

It is a form of support, and preferable to ending up on the streets or in prison, but it openly rejects science and evidence-based pharmacology. For the first time in this country, experts say psychiatry's critics are mounting a sustained broadly based effort to provide people with practical options rather than alleging abuses like overmedication and involuntary restraint.[133] Such programs are said to be proliferating now … because of society's shameful neglect of the severely ill … which creates a vacuum of great need (but blaming society is misplaced). Therapy psychiatrists are dispensing psychoanalytic psychotherapy, which absorbs most of their office time.

If they were skilled pharmacologists, they could treat ten times the number of patients—and there might not be a need for HVN at all because they'd be practicing like all other medical specialists rather than being philosophers at leisure.

The article states that about three quarters of people on medication for psychosis stop taking it in eighteen months. Is this true of any other medical specialty? (In the case of psychiatry, I am using the words ***medical specialty*** very loosely). Do 75 percent of patients of cardiologists, internists, rheumatologists stop their medications in eighteen months?

In this country, there is very little collaboration between HVN and

---

[133] Ibid.

similar organizations and psychiatry. As Gail Hornstein, a professor of psychology at Mount Holyoke College and a founding figure at HVN, states, “We need to be very careful that these groups do not become medicalized in any way.”

(What if she was speaking about people with epilepsy, cardiovascular disease, multiple sclerosis, or rheumatoid arthritis?)

Schizophrenia Is Not a Brain Disorder

Psychiatry, because of its nonmedical inclinations and reputation, erodes its credibility that it adheres to evidence-based practice (using scientific studies to support clinical decision-making). Quite frankly, most do not. A grievous side effect (and there is no other specialty of medicine that suffers from it) is every opinion goes. Everyone is an expert.

One such expert is Tyler Mostul. In an article exploring mental health,[134] he cites no fewer than seventy references. Any layperson would easily think it’s a medical document of some authority, especially individuals with prodromal or incipient schizophrenia! Yes, indeed, schizophrenia is not a brain disorder! (So, who needs evidence-based treatment?)

He sets out immediately—employing references from literature throughout his document—that schizophrenia does not have biological causes. He states traditional medical researchers claim that the brains of people with schizophrenia have common pathological features, but in reality, all schizophrenic brains are different.

Another logical flaw is that traditional researchers completely ignore the importance of external events, forgetting that the brain is designed to respond to its environment. One of those external events is the prescription of antipsychotic medications that change brain chemistry.

When it was discovered antipsychotic medications block the

[134] “Exploring Mental Health; Schizophrenia: Not a Brain Disorder.” December 20, 2015.

dopamine DO receptor, psychiatry quickly jumped to the conclusion that schizophrenia is caused by a chemical imbalance, which antipsychotic medications cure by reducing overstimulation of dopamine receptors.

But then it was discovered that the drugs, while initially blocking the dopamine system, cause a rebound that the brain compensates for, providing even more dopamine and a greater sensitivity to that neurotransmitter. The net result is the drugs meant to control dopamine lead to a paradoxical increase in it, which requires still higher doses of antipsychotic medications to control.

> In reality, several reviewers have confirmed there are no consistent differences in dopamine activity between drug-free people with schizophrenia and people without the disease. Psychiatry has failed to prove that a dopaminergic (chemical imbalance) plays any role in the symptoms of schizophrenia, but they continue to advance the theory, because without it, biological psychiatry could no longer justify use of antipsychotics and instead would have to admit that they are simply mind-numbing medications that may relieve some symptoms but do not cure anything.[135]

In the longer term, they aggravate psychosis, worsen symptoms, and cause permanent side effects such as tardive dyskinesia or tardive psychosis, which can only be suppressed by raising doses even higher.

(Mr. Mostul does not describe the symptoms of tardive dyskinesia, but it can be a disfiguring neurological illness. The antidote is having an experienced pharmacologically oriented psychiatrist who carefully monitors patients for incipient side effects.)

> Biological psychiatry also claims the brains of schizophrenics have larger ventricles, which is the

---

135 New York Times, 2008–2011.

> cause. They take this as incontestable evidence. However, psychiatric medications cause reduction in the brain volume and increase in ventricles.

This includes six references. Mostul refers to what he terms is one of the largest MRI studies to date in the *Archives of General Psychiatry*, in which it was reported, "The more drugs you've been given, the more brain volume you lose. The prefrontal cortex doesn't get the input it needs and is being shut down by drugs. That reduces psychotic symptoms. It also causes the prefrontal cortex to slowly atrophy."[136]

In summary, to continue to claim schizophrenia is a chronic brain disorder caused by enlarged ventricles, less gray matter, and less white matter in the brain … without citing evidence is irresponsible, and at its worst negligent. Mainstream psychiatry's claims that biological mechanisms are causes of schizophrenia is unfounded, and standard psychiatric treatment regimens based on unproven causal theories are largely unwarranted.

You have heard from Mr. Mostul; now, let's review the findings of researchers across America who are striving to understand the causes of schizophrenia.

As you make your way through this extensive accumulation of scientifically derived data, deliberately presented in some detail, ask yourself, if schizophrenia is really a mental health problem or a complex (physical) brain disease—as physical as neurological diseases such as epilepsy, multiple sclerosis or amyolateral sclerosis. The author, not being a neuroscientist, has attempted to simplify the information in the following article, but by all means obtain the original.[137]

The authors of this detailed, comprehensive article ask when the symptoms of schizophrenia first appear—at the time of the first psychotic episode (which is a very obvious symptomatic stage) or

---

[136] New York Times, 2008–2011.

[137] "The Neurobiology and Treatment of First Episode Schizophrenia," Kahn, R. S., Sommer, L. E. Molecular *Psychiatry*, Feb. 2015, 84–97. Published online, July 22, 2014. doi: 10.1038/m0.2014, 66.

long before that, when the symptoms are much more subtle, but nevertheless reflect ongoing neurobiological pathological changes in the brain?

The researchers first addressed a critical issue from the point of view of making a timely diagnosis and initiating effective treatment to avoid progression of the disease. Should this occur at the time of the appearance of psychotic symptoms, which generally are fairly obvious to observers—or far earlier?

In the current mental health care system, diagnosis always occurs with the onset of gross psychotic symptoms. Even then, if the patient lucks out by being treated by a decent provider, 75–80 percent will respond to competently prescribed antipsychotic medication.

Unfortunately, however, the treatment is so scattered and inconsistent that the majority relapse. The recovery rate from a relapse is dramatically lower, around 17 percent. Optimal treatment requires consistency experience, good clinical judgment, and educational efforts by the provider, so the patient continues treatment as recommended. Otherwise, the course of the disease results in deterioration of personality, decrements in functioning, disabilities, revolving-door hospitalizations, poverty, jail time, and often homelessness.

Unfortunately, the neurobiological pathological processes in the brain have started up to a decade before the first psychotic episode, unrecognized in the current mental health care system, and therefore untreated.

The onset of the disease occurs in early puberty, with the appearance of cognitive symptoms. Brain growth is stunted starting before age thirteen (and long before any medications have been prescribed.) Intracranial volume is reduced. Particularly apparent is loss of gray matter, mainly expressed as reductions in cortical thickness. White matter in never-medicated patients shows axonal and glial damage.

The gray matter deficits are most prominent in the frontal and temporal cortices. The cortical thinning pathology continues after the first psychotic episode absent effective treatment.

The loss of gray matter is correlated with cognitive and clinical outcomes. Cognitive symptoms, though less obvious than psychotic symptoms, are nevertheless real and associated with encroaching difficulties of development and functioning.

Unfortunately, hardly any mental health professionals, including therapy psychiatrists, have any understanding or recognition of cognitive symptoms and certainly not any idea of the associated neurobiological brain pathological processes. Cognitive symptoms often begin subtly and progress slowly.

Symptoms include impaired judgment and decision-making, loss of short-term or long-term memory, impairments in motor coordination, and emotional stability.

GABA Metabolism-Glial Cell Participation

As symptoms progress, there is a reduction in control over one's actions and degradation of learning, memory, perception, and problem-solving. There are three major pathological mechanisms associated with gray matter loss: pathology of the dopaminergic neurotransmission system, hypofunction of the N-methyl-D-aspartate receptor, and increased inflammation processes in the brain.

In working out these pathological mechanisms, neuroimaging studies have been performed on more than eighteen thousand affected individuals, including 771 who have never taken medication.

Dopaminergic Dysregulation

Recent positron-emission tomography studies (PET) indicate in never-medicated patients, there is increased dopamine synthesis and more rapid turnover in the striatum. There is preliminary evidence of increases of postsynaptic striatal dopamine receptors.

The increased dopaminergic neurotransmission is the final common pathway to psychotic symptoms, but this mechanism does not operate in isolation.

N-Methyl-D-Aspartate Receptor Hypofunction (NMDAr)

This mechanism plays a role in the early onset of cognitive symptoms (long before the onset of psychosis). Poor functioning of the NMDAr receptor results in reduced GABA-ergic neurotransmission, which results in insufficient inhibition of secondary glutamatergic (excitatory) neurons that fire with greater frequency and intensity, and by innervating dopaminergic neurons, provoke their excessive firing in the mesolimbic pathway.

This mechanism is associated with well-known risk genes for schizophrenia, such as DISC-1, dysbindin, SHANK, and NRG-1, which influence glutamatergic neurotransmission. Postmortem studies consistently demonstrate a decrease in an important subpopulation of GABA-interneurons in the brains of people with schizophrenia. NMDA is also involved in brain development, for example, of the prefrontal cortex and hippocampus.

Increased Pro-Inflammatory Status

The third mechanism likely underlying the signs and symptoms of schizophrenia is increased inflammatory processes in the brain. Postmortem studies of the brains of individuals with schizophrenia demonstrate signs of low-grade chronic inflammation.

Epidemiological studies consistently show that following infections, viral or bacteriological, there is a significant increased risk of developing schizophrenia. A recent study demonstrated 10 percent of people with schizophrenia have antibodies to the NMDAr versus only .4 percent of controls.

Three genome-wide association studies in 2009 demonstrate increased levels of MHC class-1 inflammatory molecules. The main immune cells of the developing, immature brain are microglia. Two studies using 11C-PK11195 PET imaging demonstrated increased levels of activation of these cells in the temporal lobes early in the course of schizophrenia versus controls. When they become activated, they abandon their neurotrophic functions such as guiding axons, producing neurotrophins like BDNF, leaving neurons in suboptimal condition, and instead produce several neurotoxic substances, such as free radicals and proinflammatory cytokines, which damage neurons and glial cells, resulting in brain volume loss and cognitive dysfunction (again, long before the onset of psychosis).

Also, excess glutamate is produced, which the hypofunctioning NMDAr fails to neutralize as it should. The cytokines, especially IL-6, which are induced by the inflammatory state, also lead to the production of superoxides, additional toxic molecules.

The progression of inflammatory processes worsens the hypofunction of the NMDAr by means of altered tryptophan catabolism, which also in response to inflammatory processes, stops producing its end product, serotonin, and substitutes kynurenic acid, which also inhibits NMDAr at its glycine site. Several studies show increased levels of kynurenic acid versus controls.

It is obvious the inflammatory processes are self-compounding and progressive. It is critical to get ahead of them by diagnosing and treating them early in the disease—long before the breakout of psychotic symptomatology.

The Consensus of Researchers

The operation of these three pathophysiological mechanisms may vary in different individuals with schizophrenia. About a third demonstrate increased inflammatory status of the brain with increased serum immunity markers.

It is hoped future research will shed further light on: further elucidating dopaminergic pathology, NMDAr hypofunction, and pro-inflammatory mechanisms.

They all agree it is critical, particularly for the future millions who will be at genetic risk for schizophrenia, to diagnose and treat the illness long before the outbreak of obvious psychotic symptoms.

Treatment of Schizophrenia

To date, treatment has been focused solely on the late stage of the disease with the appearance of clear-cut, obvious psychotic symptoms, and that form of treatment, with antipsychotic medication, even now, the application and implementation of these treatments is far from optimal.[138] This is because of the moth-eaten, fragmented treatment currently occurring in the so-called mental health care system by a polyglot assortment of grossly ill-equipped therapists, counselors, and therapy psychiatrists, ill-prepared, except for rare exceptions, to provide appropriate, consistent treatment for this progressive brain disease.

Psychiatry (again, with rare exceptions) is the only medical specialty that is basically ignorant of the operations of the one organ, the brain, they are responsible for. (It's as if a surgeon during chest surgery does not know what the vagus nerve is—let alone where it is!)

Totally lacking in the current mental health care system is the ability to detect and treat the disease in its early stages, before brain damage has become permanent. The symptoms of the early stage disease are subtler, requiring skilled expertise to recognize, understand, and treat.

There are potentially new treatments on the horizon that may halt the disease process early on—if they are started and used proactively. The common thread is that they must be started long before the onset of obvious psychotic symptoms.

Glutamatergic Treatments

Modulation of the glycine transporter, for example, with a molecule termed sarcosine, has demonstrated some improvement in cognitive and negative symptoms, and may have much more benefit if utilized in early-stage disease. Two classes of selective GABA-ergic drugs have

[138] Ibid, 8.

been proposed to enhance cognition, an a5 inverse selective agonist and an A2/3 selective agonist.

There is strong evidence from animal studies that allosteric modulation of the a5 subunit of the GABA-A receptor can lead to improvements in cognition in early-stage disease. Such glutamatergic and/or GABA-ergic medications, to emphasize again, must be given early on, before the window of opportunity has closed.[139] (That is long before the onset of psychotic symptoms.)

Anti-Inflammatory Agents

A recent meta-analysis of studies has shown that aspirin, n-acetylcysteine (NAC), and estrogens (in women) may have efficacy in schizophrenia. Another study did show polyunsaturated fatty acids significantly reduced or delayed transition to psychosis. After eight weeks, there was a significant drop in negative symptoms, and there were higher scores in global functioning at twelve weeks.

As is the case for glutamatergic treatments, anti-inflammatories are less effective by the time psychotic symptoms have occurred, which is indicative of irreversible damage to neurons and glia cells reflected in brain volume loss, which has been repeatedly demonstrated with magnetic resonance imaging studies. One anti-inflammatory imaging agent, NAC, may be of particular interest if utilized early in the course of the disease. It targets a diverse array of factors, including glutamatergic neurotransmission, the antioxidant, glutathione, neurotrophins, apoptosis, mitochondrial function, and inflammatory pathways. It has a benign side effect profile, and it can prevent brain volume loss, cognitive deterioration, and subsequent transition to psychosis.

Interestingly, exercise, if employed in early stage disease, may in conjunction with pharmacology, alleviate progressive loss of gray matter.

Another potential nonmedicinal intervention is repetitive

---

[139] Ibid.

transcranial magnetic stimulation, which may improve GABA-ergic neurotransmission if utilized in early-stage disease by targeting specific brain regions like the dorsolateral prefrontal cortex to improve cognitive function and working memory.

In summary, at the time of first psychotic symptoms, neurobiological processes underlying schizophrenia have already been ongoing for many years. Although increased DA synthesis may be the final common pathway to psychosis, hypofunction of the NMDAr, associated decreased GABA-ergic signaling and increased pro-inflammatory status of the brain may be important mechanisms underlying cognitive dysfunction.

The contribution of these pathophysiological pathways to the clinical picture of schizophrenia mostly likely varies per individual. If we aim to intervene before the window of opportunity is closed and deviations in the brain have become hardwired, it will be key to include cognitive deterioration in the diagnosis of schizophrenia instead of postponing diagnosis until the onset of psychotic symptoms many years later.[140]

Bipolar Disorder

DUB is an acronym used in the article, "Meta-Analysis of the Interval between the Onset and Management of Bipolar Disorder."[141] It stands for *duration of untreated bipolar disorder.*

The intent of this study was to determine the actual length between the onset of the symptoms of bipolar disorder and the initiation of disease appropriate treatment. They analyzed fifty-one samples from 9,415 patients. Their final estimation was it took 5.8 years.

Can you imagine waiting six years before receiving a diagnosis for a heart attack or a seizure?

They accurately describe bipolar disorder as a debilitating illness characterized by distressing and disruptive symptoms. In the current

---

140 Ibid.

141 Dagani, Jessica, et al, *The Canadian Journal of Psychiatry*, 2016.

mental health care system, only after the disease has progressed to the stage of intense symptomatology, debilitation, and disabilities, does it have any chance of being diagnosed accurately and treated with disease-specific remedies.

(It's like waiting for the spot on a lung to expand in the lung and spread to the rest of the body before recognizing and treating it. By then, it's usually fatal.)

There is a roster of reasons the current mental health care system and therapy psychiatry function so poorly and fail the poor souls who—through no fault of their own—have bipolar disorder. The current mental health care system and its mental health providers are ill-equipped to diagnose and treat a progressive (physical) brain illness. Many have good intentions—therapists, counselors, and some therapy psychiatrists—but completely lack appropriate training, experience, and medical and pharmacological skills at the appropriate professional level. The list of deficiencies is long and ultimately leads to tragic results because the main hope of the sufferers is that an appropriate diagnosis is made early in the course of the disease so appropriate treatments prevent its progression!

1. If a bipolar patient is referred for mental health treatment, often that involves nonspecialists and poorly coordinated services.
2. In the first year of the illness, less than 20 percent even receive an appropriate diagnosis.
3. Inexperienced therapists/clinicians are unaware that bipolar disorder can present first solely with depression, and they miss the diagnosis entirely. They lack the clinical skills to diagnose hypomania, don't understand the course of the disease, and do not identify when it had its onset. They are ignorant of the skills needed to conduct specific interviewing approaches for bipolar disorder, including the cross-sectional clinical interview utilizing life charting.

4. They attribute presenting symptoms to other conditions like unipolar depression, ADHD, and personality disorders; they lack knowledge of the stages of illness requiring stage specific interventions; they fail to consider longitudinal and corroborative information to make an accurate diagnosis; and they don't want to make the diagnosis because it means long-term treatment would be necessary, and it will be stigmatizing (particularly in the case of adolescents and young adults).

So, the disease just progresses, battering brains as it goes! What's the difference if it isn't diagnosed on a timely basis? It's only a mental health problem! If these people wanted to, they could snap themselves out of it! It's mental health problem that requires specific physical treatments—no less than uncontrolled seizures—and the treatments are nearly identical (with anticonvulsants except for lithium). The same anticonvulsants are used to treat seizures—except people with epilepsy don't have to wait six years before treatment starts!

So, what is to be done about DUB? Who is going to do it? How much longer will we (and the sufferers) have to wait? Let us pray. But prayer is best supplemented by action! Action must be taken by all of us concerned with the gross deficiencies of the psychiatrists' mental health care system since they will be the greatest obstacle to true progress.

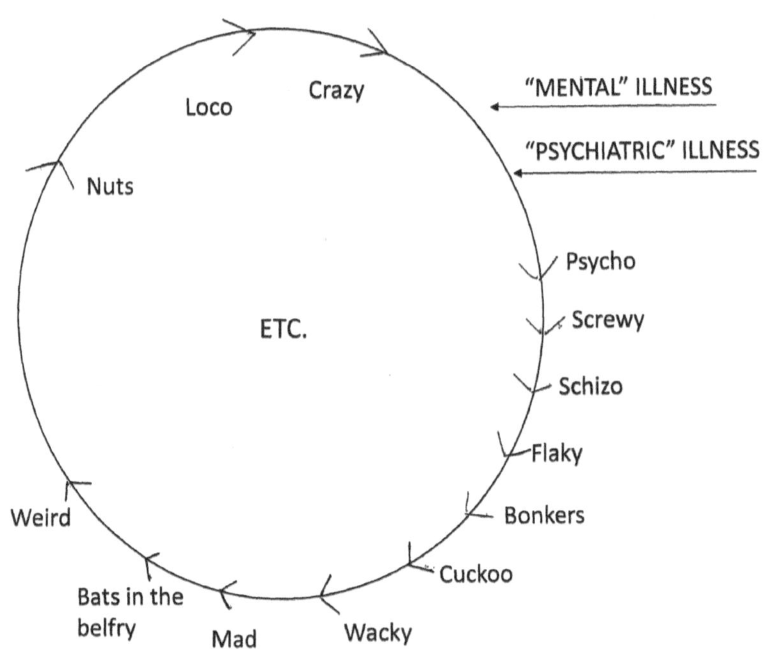

Stigma

As long as the treacherous dichotomy exists in our thoughts, media, and institutions, there will always be stigma. The mental labeling of the illnesses being discussed here will not be disentangled from stigmatizing, stereotyped thinking until they are systematically and authoritatively reclassified as physical brain disorders—and the era of mental health disorders and mental health treatment is completely expunged both from our conscious and unconscious thinking!

Gabriel Gerlingen et al. set out to perform a systematic review of stigma toward the mentally ill and the impact on them.[142] They analyzed fifty-four studies with 5,871 patients recruited form all types of health care facilities, from rural and urban environments, who were in all stages of severity of disease.

They used two definitions of stigma, that of Goffman, that stigma is an attribute that is deeply discrediting and reduces the person who bears it from a whole and usual person to a tainted discounted one or of Link and Phelan, as the occurrence of labeling, stereotyping, separation, status loss, and discrimination. They distinguish between two basic categories of stigma: public stigma and personal stigma.

Public stigma focuses on public concepts of mental illness and the negative reactions toward mentally ill individuals displayed by individuals or societal groups. Personal stigma refers to how the stigmatized individual internalizes the negative beliefs of stigmatization, accompanied by the diminishment of positive beliefs about the self, in turn yielding negative consequences: 87 percent reported feeling stigmatized in interpersonal interactions, and 64.5 percent felt more generalized stigmatization. They identified the correlates of stigmatization, including its impact on outcomes.

Personal Stigma as Predictor of Outcome

Perceived/experienced stigma was found to predict higher depression, more social anxiety, more secrecy, and more withdrawal as coping strategies, along with lower quality of life, lower self-efficacy, lower self-esteem, lower social functioning, less support, and less mastery. Self-stigma predicted more depression, more social anxiety, lower quality of life, less self-esteem, less social functioning, less hope, less vocational functioning, less recovery, less support, and less treatment compliance.

So, what's to be done about stigma? Who is going to do it? How much longer will we—and the sufferers—have to wait? Let us pray.

---

142 "Personal stigma in schizophrenia spectrum disorders: a systematic review of prevalence rates, correlates, impact and interventions," *World Psychiatry,* June 2013; 12 (2): 155–164.

GLOSSARY

axon. A long, slender projection of a nerve cell or neuron that conducts nerve impulses to other neurons.

dendrite. Branched projections from a neuron that receives impulses from other neurons, which are transmitted to the cell body.

dendritic spines (enrichment). A small membranous protrusion from a neuron's dendrites that receive input from a single axon at a synapse. The dendrites of one neuron can contain thousands of spines. They may play a role in memory, and the more contacts with other neurons, the better.

dorsolateral-prefrontal cortex. An area of the prefrontal cortex, which is one of the most recently evolved. Important functions are executive functions such as planning, cognitive flexibility, abstract reasoning, and organizational capabilities. It, however, requires connectedness to other faciliatory brain areas.

glucocorticoid receptor. A receptor to which cortisol and other glucocorticoids bind. The glucocorticoid system functions as a major component and influence on the endocrine system, particularly the stress response, and plays a major role in MDD and PTSD.

hippocampus. There are two. They are part of the limbic system. They play a role in the consolidation of memory from short to long term, as well as spatial navigation.

hypothalamic-pituitary-adrenal axis (HPA). A complex set of interactions between three endocrine (hormone) glands, the hypothalamus, the pituitary gland, and the adrenal gland. It controls the stress response and is involved in the neurobiology of many psychiatric disorders, including MDD, bipolar disorder, anxiety disorders, irritable bowel syndrome, fibromyalgia, and alcoholism.

neural plasticity. The capacity of neural tissue to adopt to internal and external stressors.

neurogenesis. The process by which neurons are generated from neural stem cells. These cells give rise to all the neurons in the brain.

nucleotides. Organic molecules that are subunits of DNA and RNA, the hereditary molecules.

promotor region of genes. A region of the DNA molecule that initiates transcription (duplication) of that particular gene. The initiation of transcription is a multistep process involving several mechanisms.

SNP. A variation in a single nucleotide that is located in a specific position in the genome. They underlie differences in the susceptibility to disease.

striatum. A subcortical part of the forebrain and a critical part of the reward system. It receives glutamatergic and dopaminergic inputs from different sources and is the primary input into the basal ganglia system. It coordinates multiple aspects of cognition, including motor and action planning, decision-making, motivation, reinforcement, and reward perception.

CHAPTER 26

Latest Developments

The therapy psychiatrists have just held their latest convention. There was a rigorous debate whether deep emotional conflicts in the id and superego could be associated with physical genes. The assembly converged on a consensus that by the very nature of deep emotional conflicts, riddled with complexity, shifting emotions, and battling forces, they could not possibly be a product of such single tiny physical genes, but rather of far more complexly constructed mental genes. There was agreement to raise dues for the purpose of initiating a broad research effort to locate them. There was a research suggestion that mental genes might be—by virtue of the inherent complexity—a form of holographic phenomenon.

The assembly also issued a declaration about the abysmal direction so-called scientific research is taking the field. "They are turning the field into a dismal, chaotic, incomprehensible alphabet soup." They formally list some of the strange, heterogeneous meaningless words, letters, and numbers that make no sense: Neuropeptide Y, Receptor-Y2, NPY2R, C-allele of rs6857715, polymorphisms of FKBPS, SNPs rs1360780, rs 4713916, rs 3800373, rs755658, BDNF, pro BDNF, mBDNF/pro BDNF ratio, and so forth.

To be serious, ongoing studies employing the genome-wide association techniques (GWAS) and the meta-analysis of selected high-quality studies continue to reinforce the significance of heritability for

MDD, which is now estimated at 40 percent.[143] (The other 60 percent is the outcome of the life trajectory from conception to death).

New candidate genes that increase the vulnerability are being identified and studied. One newly identified gene is for FK506 binding protein 51 (FKBP5) a hypothalamic-pituitary-adrenal (HPA) axis-related gene that alters the glucocorticoid receptor response for cortisol. It is felt the increased vulnerability to MDD by genetic factors occurs through the synergistic operation of multiple SNPs acting in concert. This entire hereditary operation is no different for mental disorders than for other complex diseases like heart disease, diabetes, or rheumatoid arthritis.

Another interesting gene associated with MDD is neuropeptide Y (NPY), which is thought to play a role in the stress response, which is so important as a major trigger for MDD. A particular variant for the neuropeptide receptor Y2 (NPY2R), promotor region of the gene may foster an abnormal stress response, for example variant rs6857715. In a study,[144] genetic analysis of 595 patients with MDD were compared to 1,295 typical, healthy control participants. Four common SNPs (rs1360780, rs4713916, rs3800373 and rs755658) were identified as more selective in patients with MDD, therefore conferring more risk for MDD. Two alleles, rs1360780T and rs3800373C, were particularly prominent.

BDNF

In general medicine, laboratory examinations of plasma levels of different body molecules are standard (sugar levels, tests of kidney function, liver function tests, counts for blood cells, etc.), The results

[143] Kranjac, Dinko, PhD, medical editor. *Psychiatry Advisor*, Sept. 11,2016. From Rao S., et al. "Common variants in FKBPS gene and major depressive disorder (MDD) susceptibility: a comprehensive meta-analysis." *Sci Rep.* 2016; 32687.

[144] Kranjac, Dinko, PhD medical editor. *Psychiatry Advisor*, September 6, 2016. From Treuflein, J. et al. « Association between neuropeptide T-receptor Y2 promotor variant rs6857715 and major depressive disorder." *Psychiatric Genetics*, 2016.

are a prime source of data for distinguishing between different disease states (differential diagnosis) and establishing levels whether normal, abnormally elevated or low).

A stark dividing line between real physical illnesses and mental illnesses has always been the absence of equivalent laboratory testing, making it an impossibility to get objective measurements of body substances. This dividing line has stood like a high wall, keeping the mental illnesses isolated and separated from real diseases of the body, a justification for discrimination against the mentally ill and a reinforcer of stigmatization.

Modern neuroscience might begin to erode this treacherous dichotomy, but we'll all have to work hard at it because the dichotomy is so entrenched in our minds at every level—unconscious, subconscious, conscious—and implanted by therapy psychiatry.

Finally, substances that play a role in serious mood illnesses, MDD and bipolar disorder, can be measured in the laboratory using blood samples. (Could they be real physical illnesses like diabetes or epilepsy?) Brain-derived neurotropic factor[145] has already been described as a very important neurotrophic molecule involved in neuronal protection and survival, the facilitation of synaptic transmission, the promotion of neural plasticity, and the enrichment of dendritic spines. Data indicate it is relevant in the symptomatic presentation of mood illnesses.

The mature form of BDNF (mBDNF) has a predecessor molecule, pro BDNF. If both are measured in the laboratory, another relevant laboratory value, the mBDNF/proBDNF ratio can be calculated. The delay to making a diagnosis of bipolar disorder in the current mental health care system is six years. If major mood disorders receive the proper attention by qualified, experienced brain psychiatrists who understand the molecular dysregulations of bipolar disorder, the diagnosis could be made in a matter of days. Patients are fortunate to

---

145 "Ratio of mBDNF to proBDNF for Differential Diagnosis of Major Depressive Disorder and Bipolar Depression." Zhao, G., Zhang, C., Chen, J. et al. *Mol. Neurobiol* (2016)

get to be evaluated and diagnosed early in the course of their illness. Bipolar disorder is distinguished from MDD and normal controls by having significantly lower mBDNF levels. Unipolar depression (MDD) is distinguished by a significantly higher ratio of mBDNF to proBDNF than bipolar patients or individuals without a mood illness.

The objective of "The Neuroanatomy of and Cognitive Deficits in Depression"[146] was to identify brain areas involved in contributing to the symptomatic picture of MDD. They identified multiple sites that underlie the pathogenesis of MDD. There is a long list: amygdalae, hippocampus, prefrontal cortex, anterior cingulate cortex, striatum, nucleus accumbens, the thalamus, and the dorsolateral prefrontal cortex.

In comparison to normal control subjects not having MDD, all these sites are smaller, reflecting a process of atrophy. For example, the hippocampus can be up to 19 percent smaller than in normal controls. The hippocampus is a vital structure involved in learning and memory. In addition to atrophy of these structures, there is evidence of aberrant neural activity and alterations of neural circuits. The atrophy of the hippocampus does not precede the onset of MDD, but it is a consequence of the ongoing untreated disease process in which the number of untreated days of depression is directly proportional to the degree of atrophy and the abnormalities of synapses in the hippocampus.

Antidepressant medications promote neurogenesis in the hippocampus, as do adjunctive therapies like CBT. However, the more severe the major depression, the greater the need for sophisticated pharmacological therapy.

During the active disease state, the metabolic activity of the dorsolateral prefrontal cortex (DLPFC) is abnormally low. Like the hippocampus, the DLPFC is a vital center for maintaining higher cognitive functions like working memory, cognitive flexibility,

---

[146] *Psychiatry Advisor*; Kranjac, Dinko, PhD, medical editor, Sept. 2, 2016. "A Review of the Neuroanatomy of Depression," Oake, Peter, et al, DOI: 10. 1002/ ca. 22–181.

adequate attention abilities, and motivational drive. In response to appropriate antidepressant pharmacological treatment, there is a significant improvement of the functions of the DLPFC.

Again, this study is an additional strong confirmation that the major mood illnesses are not mere mental health problems but complex (physical) brain diseases.

CHAPTER 27

Final Words

Exciting things are being discovered by therapy-psychiatry researchers. They have learned there are mental genes that are causative of mental illnesses, which are located in the id and superego. These genes precipitate the unconscious conflicts deeply buried there. A critical question for future research is how the genes can be therapeutically reregulated by the skilled use of psychodynamically concise interpretations by the psychiatrist during the course of psychoanalytically oriented psychotherapy, to target specific conflicts. In the future, it may be possible to alter mental genes, reducing the total time needed for an analysis by several months.

Let's get serious. It is tragic when a young person with schizophrenia does not find appropriate treatment for years after the disease onset, usually only at the time the symptoms of the disease have progressed to the chronic stage, causing incapacitating symptoms and the demolishment of that individual's chances of leading a normal life with reasonable achievements and happiness.

Early-stage treatments already exist and are being further developed, but on the practical, clinical, and systemic level in the current mental health care system, it is the rare patient who has access to them. It would be so much more merciful to nip schizophrenia in the bud, permitting an individual to lead a normal life, than to let the disease fester and progress as it does now. That would require the disease be diagnosed far earlier than currently—on average ten years earlier—long before psychotic symptoms become apparent. It needs to happen at the time of onset of the more subtle cognitive symptoms.

The specialty of neurology also diagnoses and treats brain diseases. Usually, when neurological symptoms first occur, most patients and their families automatically understand the symptoms are manifestations of a physical disease process. They immediately consult with a family doctor who will refer to a neurologist—or they independently consult with a neurologist. They do not spend the first ten years of their diseases going to physical therapists with absolutely no input from the appropriate medical specialist, the neurologist.

The Importance of Early Intervention

Best is primary prevention, the attempt to prevent a disease before its onset. Public health measures and prophylactic interventions are utilized. Next best is secondary prevention. The objective is to reduce the impact of a disease as early as possible in its course. Tertiary prevention aims to reduce the impact of an illness, its symptomatic burden, and any associated disabilities throughout the course of the illness.

Focusing on schizophrenia, the current mental health care system fails at every level. Schizophrenia is far advanced and disabling before some of the affected received appropriate treatment.

What is to be done? How can people early in the course of schizophrenia get to be evaluated and treated on a timely basis with appropriate treatments. This can never occur in the current mental health care system, which should be obvious from previous discussions. A purely medicalized approach—similar to how neurological diseases are treated in the medical system, with some tweaks—will be mandatory. Just as neurological diseases are automatically assumed to be physical, so must be the so-called psychiatric diseases. The first priority, if there is to be effective reform, is to reframe the terminology. Referencing them as *mental* must be eliminated. Many readers are so habituated to the treacherous dichotomy that human diseases are categorized either as physical or mental. This would appear to be a totally unrealistic objective, but it is critical. The mental framework automatically dredges up the dark garbage of stigma, shame, and ghostly stereotypes. There is an alternative terminology, which will not be an obstacle to all three levels of prevention.

The neurologist, in the medical system, does not spend forty-five-minutes talking to a given patient every week. Therefore, he can provide his expertise to a far larger assemblage of patients than the therapy psychiatrist. And the neurologist is a true physician; he knows the brain, its structure, its mechanisms, and its pathologies. He has learned in depth about that physical organ and has expertise in specific pharmacological and other treatment modalities that speak to the physical pathologies. The neurologist refers to nonmedical specialists to provide patients additional therapeutic assistance *after* a thorough neurological evaluation.

I have repeatedly used the terminology *brain psychiatrist* in this discussion. To review what's meant by this, he also is a true medical specialist whose practice parallels that of the neurologist in many ways. He has a formal understanding of the neurobiological brain dysregulation associated with symptoms. He would not indulge in providing forty-five-minute weekly sessions of so-called psychodynamic psychotherapy. He would refer to certified non-MD psychotherapists instead for cognitive therapies, specific behavioral therapies, group therapy, addiction-related therapies, and so forth.

There would be some tweaks from neurology. Because the psychiatric disorders have a closer association to emotional, cognitive, and behavioral dysregulations overall than neurological illnesses, the treatment sessions should be extended to twenty-five or thirty minutes. The ten-minute session—an invention of insurance companies to increase profits—is self-defeating, short-circuiting assessing and coping with stresses or necessary educational discussion focusing on the nature of symptoms and the details of specific treatments. The initial evaluation must never be shorter than an hour!

And the nomenclature must change. There will be no transitioning to more timely and efficacious diagnosis and treatment without a new terminology. The root, *neuro*, as in neurology is of Greek origin, meaning *nerve*. It pertains to a nerve, or nerves, or the nervous system. The root *psych* as in *psychotic*, has a much more recent origin. It is a variant of *psycho*. It originated in student slang in 1895.[147] Obviously the pedigrees are starkly different. It would seem easy enough to adopt the root *neuro*. That would imply these disorders are also biologically based. Hence, *neuriatry, neuriatrist*, and *neuropharmacology*.

There is an overabundance of mental disorders listed in *The Diagnostic and Statistical Manual of Mental Disorders*. All of these should be reclassified as emotional, cognitive, behavioral, and personality dysregulations—not mental problems. The *DSM-5* should be eliminated, and all neuriatric disorders and the various dysregulation only listed in ICD-10-CM, along with all the other physical illnesses and symptoms, and not kept isolated in a separate mental category.

How neuriatrists are trained is a critical issue. They must know the brain! And they must practice in the medical system, like neurologists. This will only happen with the help of a growing awareness on the part of patients, families, and legislators. We will have to push for these changes against the resistance of organized psychiatry.

---

[147] *The Dictionary of American Slang*, fourth edition by Kipfer, B. A., Chapman, Robert L., PhD, 2007.

www.ingramcontent.com/pod-product-compliance
Lightning Source LLC
Chambersburg PA
CBHW031818170526
45157CB00001B/109

* 9 7 8 1 4 8 0 8 7 2 0 8 0 *